NURSING THE IMAGE

Ideas of nursing and nurses carry a powerful social charge. The image of the nurse continues to be a symbol of caring and of duty at the same time as it projects a view of femininity, 'stereotypical' in its gender relations. *Nursing the Image* traces how differences of gender, race and class amongst nurses have challenged traditional concepts of professional identity and irrevocably changed nursing's image.

Uniquely, this book argues that nursing's professional identity in post-war Britain is a discourse of white femininity that women actively construct and practise in conditions and circumstances not of their choosing. Images of nursing in the media and promotional recruitment literature are juxta-posed with written and oral accounts of becoming a nurse gathered from a diverse group of women. These auto/biographies reveal how a Victorian legacy of white middle-class values, inherited from Florence Nightingale's pioneering efforts to make nursing a respectable profession for women, permeated nursing's professional identity and shaped nurses' attitudes to their working lives. For those deemed 'unsuitable' for training because of their gender, class or skin colour, many of whom arrived in England from Britain's former colonies to staff the newly created National Health Service, the 'angel' embodied an outdated system of values and practices that had to be challenged.

Julia Hallam provides a unique record of popular culture's negotiation of female identity during a period of rapid modernisation and change. She explores a modern myth of femininity, extending our understanding of the ways in which women adopt, adapt and resist dominant conceptions of femininity even as they engage in its everyday practices. *Nursing the Image* will be a valuable source for any courses dealing with the social history of nursing, the understanding of health, and women and gender studies, and for sociology courses focusing on the cultural or gendered study of health.

Julia Hallam is Director of English and Communication Studies, University of Liverpool.

NURSING THE IMAGE

Media, culture and professional identity

Julia Hallam

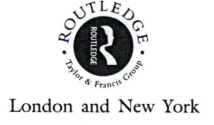

London and New York

First published 2000
by Routledge
2 Park Square, Milton Park, Abingdon, Oxon, OX14 4RN

Simultaneously published in the USA and Canada
by Routledge
270 Madison Ave, New York NY 10016

Routledge is an imprint of the Taylor & Francis Group

Transferred to Digital Printing 2009

Typeset in Galliard by
Florence Production Ltd, Stoodleigh, Devon

British Library Cataloguing in Publication Data
A catalogue record for this book is available from the British Library

Library of Congress Cataloging-in-Publication Data
Hallam, Julia, 1952–
Nursing the image : media, culture, and professional identity / Julia Hallam
p. ; cm.
Includes bibliographical references and index.
1. Nurses–Great Britain–Public opinion. 2. Public opinion–Great Britain. 3.
Nurses–Great Britain–Psychology. 4. Sex role–Great Britain. 5. Professional
socialization–Great Britain. 6. Nursing–Social aspects–Great Britain. 7. Feminist
theory. I. Title.
[DNLM: 1. Nurses–Great Britain. 2. Feminism–Great Britain. 3. Prejudice–Great
Britain. 4. Social Perception–Great Britain. 5. Stereotyping–Great Britian. WY 16
H182n 2000]
RT82.H348 2000
610.73′0941–dc21

ISBN 0–415–18455–X (pbk)
ISBN 0–415–18454–1 (hbk)

Publisher's Note

For my sister Vicky

CONTENTS

ACKNOWLEDGEMENTS

This book has had a long gestation and many people have contributed to the ideas, information and materials that constitute its substance. A major influence during my early years in nursing was Sister Mary Edwards at the David Lewis Northern Hospital in Liverpool. Her wisdom and healing skills taught me that there was far more to nursing than being a 'good girl' and I thank her for her fortitude and strength of mind. The women like her who trained me are the subjects of this book; for those who allowed me to question them about their nursing lives, I am deeply grateful. Special thanks to the ten women who, by their request, remain anonymous; their thoughts on how our identities as nurses were nurtured and developed are woven throughout the text. Thanks to Anne Marie Rafferty (London) and Judith Parker (Melbourne) for their enthusiasm and encouragement, and colleagues who attended the Nottingham conference in 1995, Nursing History and the Politics of Welfare.

Terry Lovell, Richard Dyer, Sheila Campbell and Annecke Marshall at the University of Warwick provided support and inspiration in the early days. Elizabeth Wilson and Jackie Stacey commented on an initial draft of the text. Heather Hoëpfl, Alice Kiger, Christine Knox, Marion McMahon, Nickianne Moody and Deborah Philips have shared their ideas and brought source materials to my attention. My colleagues at Liverpool University, John Corner, Kay Richardson and Maggie Scammell, created the collegiate atmosphere of generosity and support that enabled me to finish the writing; Edwina Welham and staff at Routledge have safely steered the project through its final stages. Thank you all for your help in bringing this project to fruition.

LIST OF ILLUSTRATIONS

ILLUSTRATION
ACKNOWLEDGEMENTS

Thanks to staff at Central Library, Liverpool, the Royal College of Nursing archive and the National Film Archive for help with locating recruitment and related materials.

Thanks also to the people and institutions listed below for permission to reproduce their images. While the publishers have made every effort to contact the copyright holders of previously published material in this volume, they would be grateful to hear from any they were unable to contact.

Figure 2.1(a) Cover, *Sue Barton: Student Nurse*, Helen Dore Boylston (Knight Books, 1971)

Figure 2.1(b) Cover, *Sue Barton: Superintendent Nurse*, Helen Dore Boylston (Knight Books, 1981)

Figure 2.2 Cover, *Cherry Ames: Night Supervisor*, Julie Tatham (World Distributors, 1961). Reproduced by kind permission of Robert Wells.

Figure 2.3 Publicity poster for *The Feminine Touch* (dir. Pat Jackson, 1956; adapted from the American novel *A Lamp is Heavy* by Sheila Mackay Russell and released in the USA with that title). Reproduced by kind permission of Canal+ Image UK.

Figure 2.4 Cover, *The Lambs*, Kate Norway (Mills & Boon®, 1965). Permission to reproduce cover kindly granted by Harlequin Mills & Boon® Limited.

Figure 2.5 Cover, *Junior Pro*, Kate Norway (Corgi 1974; first published by Mills & Boon®, 1959). Permission to reproduce cover kindly granted by Renee Brown. Photographer: Beverly Lebarrow. RJB Photo Library (tel. +44 (0)20 7386 7214).

Figure 3.1 Recruitment leaflet *Your Chance*, 1950s (Ministry of Labour/ Central Office of Information). By kind permission of Her Majesty's Stationery Office.

Figure 3.2 Recruitment leaflet *Nursing Today*, 1960s (Nursing Recruitment Service, King Edward's Hospital Fund). Reproduced by kind permission of King Edward's Hospital Fund.

ILLUSTRATION ACKNOWLEDGEMENTS

Figures 3.3(a) and 3.3(b) 'Classical' and 'popular' 1960s recruitment leaflets (Ministry of Labour/Ministry of Health/Central Office of Information). By kind permission of Her Majesty's Stationery Office.

Figures 3.4(a), 3.4(b) and 3.4(c) *SRN* brochure, 1960s (Ministry of Labour/Ministry of Health/Central Office of Information). By kind permission of Her Majesty's Stationery Office.

Figures 3.5(a), 3.5(b) and 3.5(c) *Proud Badge of Service*, SEN brochure, 1960s (Ministry of Labour/Ministry of Health/Central Office of Information). By kind permission of Her Majesty's Stationery Office.

Figure 3.6 *He's Stepping out in a Career that's Different*, late 1960s leaflet (Department of Health and Social Security). By kind permission of Her Majesty's Stationery Office.

Figure 3.7 *Nursing: A Profession for Men*, leaflet, 1972 (Department of Health and Social Security). By kind permission of Her Majesty's Stationery Office.

Figures 3.8(a) and 3.8(b) *Like to be Back in Nursing? Yes, it's Great to be Back* (1972) and *You'd Make a Good Nurse* (1973), leaflets (Department of Health and Social Security). By kind permission of Her Majesty's Stationery Office.

Figure 4.1(a) Cover, *One Pair of Feet*, Monica Dickens (Penguin Books, Harmondsworth: 1957). Reproduced by permission of Penguin Books Ltd. Cover illustration by Geoffrey Salter.

Figure 4.1(b) Cover, *Come Hither, Nurse*, Jane Grant (Pan Books, 1959). By kind permission of Macmillan Publishers Limited.

Figure 4.2 Nurses' Home, Liverpool, late 1950s. Photographer: Leslie Cooper, Oxton Studios, Merseyside.

INTRODUCTION

(Auto)biography, research and feminist cultural studies

> We ought to acknowledge, more honestly than we do, the
> extent to which our studies are reflections of our inner lives.
>
> (Kreiger 1991: 1)

The theoretical frameworks that shape this analysis of nursing's professional image and identity are located in feminist cultural studies, a practice that has at the centre of its concerns how texts construct knowledge of the self in relation to the social world. Analysis of films, novels and television programmes is combined with interviews, historical sources, archival materials and a range of theoretical perspectives to reveal the underlying structural relations that inform the social relations of nursing subjectivities. Cultural practices and cultural representations are part of a matrix of wider discourses that situate us as social subjects. As a researcher, I am positioned through locations such as gender, class, race, age, sexuality and geography; these socially structured and situated determinations have controlled and facilitated my access to various forms of cultural capital, and my ability to convert that capital into economic value.[1]

I became interested in the ways in which representations inscribe available subject positions on individuals when, in my mid-thirties, I first went to university in Scotland. I discovered that I was known amongst my fellow students as 'that Greenham Common woman', although I had not taken part in activities at the peace camp or envisaged myself as that 'type' of person. For young people in the mid-1980s televised images of the Greenham peace camp provided a potent symbol of feminist activism;[2] the media coverage provided a recognisable framework of interpretation in which they could locate my 'difference' as a speaking subject interested in feminism. Discursive configurations not only provide structures for understanding how we see ourselves and how others see us; they locate us in dichotomous conceptual frameworks (such as feminine/feminist, insider/outsider) and social hierarchies of difference. As a feminist researcher working in the university system, one becomes acutely aware of these hierarchies; for example, the production of medico-scientific knowledge is

1

granted higher status and receives more funding than the production of nursing knowledge. Academic disciplines situate researchers in theoretical and scholastic traditions, methodological practices and styles of writing; feminist cultural work both accepts and challenges these structures. It is often eclectic, multi-disciplinary and interdisciplinary, undertaken across a range of sites, drawing strength from a conflictual history that aims, by whatever strategic or tactical means available, to produce knowledge from an adversarial position.[3]

This project was initially motivated by a personal need to explore my own subject formation during the period I grew up and became a nurse, to examine and analyse the socio-cultural matrix in which my own subjectivity as a nurse was embedded. My childhood dilemma of 'what to do when I grow up' was clouded by a deep dread of war; born at the tail end of the 'baby boom' generation in the early 1950s, I was a Cold War child. During much of my childhood, Cold War politics generated a fear of nuclear war that created a chronic anxiety state in those around me. I grew up in an emotional climate saturated by a terror of war which I remember experiencing in three ways; indirectly through my mother's stories of her war-time experiences, directly through family and group civil defence exercises in preparation for nuclear war, and morally through a religious insistence that another war would mean the end of the world. These childhood experiences shaped my world view, my early choice of reading and, ultimately, my decision to become a nurse. I was constantly asking myself, 'what will I do if war breaks out?' and giving two answers: one solution was to run away; the other was to be brave, which meant becoming a nurse or joining the army – the two seemed to be much of a muchness at the time.

Working for the first time as an agency nurse in London in the late 1980s and experiencing the contrasts between the private sector and the underfunded National Health Service (NHS), I became acutely conscious of how both the private and public health care sectors exploit the skills of experienced nurses. Talking to women who had spent their working lives in nursing and felt, like me, that their knowledge and experience was undervalued fuelled my desire to undertake further studies. The decision to use autobiography as a method of structuring the research stemmed from an interest in exploring how experience might inform the production of knowledge. Unhappy with totalising theories that claimed women as victims of ideological positions that condemned them to suffer, I sought feminist theories that were empowering and positive about women's abilities to generate change.

Feminist academics from a range of disciplinary frameworks have become increasingly interested in the position of the researcher *vis-à-vis* the research process.[4] In the social sciences, the turn to the role of the self in constructing knowledges about the social world tends to have followed a feminist ethno-

graphic impetus that places participant observation and in-depth interviewing at the forefront of qualitative research methodologies.[5] Within this
context, an increasing self-reflexivity that locates the self as a subject artic-
ulating a particular standpoint situates interpretation as strategic intervention
that is integral to the construction of feminist knowledge (Hartsock 1987,
Harding 1991). Reacting against the dictum that researchers should present
themselves as objective, neutral and disinterested observers, feminist
researchers are often keen to reveal their personal investments in the research
process.[6] Who do feminists speak for? Who do they speak to? How can
they avoid objectification of the other, whilst still maintaining a place for
themselves? Finding a place from which to speak and write is no longer a
matter of simply adopting the language of the academic expert (Hallam
and Marshall 1993). As feminist academics, the way we use language reflects
our own relationship to and investment in the institutions in which we
find ourselves, institutions that depend on existing discursive formations to
maintain their power and authority.[7] Institutionalised discourses function
on categories of difference because difference is the essential component
of any hierarchical organisation; sharing experiences with women in similar
situations as oneself (what used to be known as 'consciousness raising')
can illuminate these differences. But perhaps, more importantly, as Carolyn
Steedman and Dorothy Smith point out, what is revealed through such
exercises is both the power and the limitations of dominant discourses to
conceptually shape and mould female identity (Steedman 1986, Smith
1988a).

Using as a basis my understanding of feminist work culled from a range
of disciplinary perspectives used in the study of film, television and popular
culture, three fields of enquiry are pursued here which tend to be treated
as discrete entities located in separate schools of thought: the popular imagination, which focuses on images of nursing in films, books and television
dramas; the professional imagination, which traces ideals of professional
identity presented in recruitment literature; and the personal imagination,
which explores the aspirations and experiences of women who became
nurses during the post-war period. In order to facilitate a socio-cultural
analysis that is historically concise and to create a framework in which it
is possible to analyse these categories and their interconnectedness, I have
concentrated on three particular 'moments' when there was a groundswell
of dense public activity featuring nursing and nurses across various texts
in a range of media forms: the late 1940s and early 1950s, the late 1950s
and early 1960s and the late 1960s to the mid-1970s. Organising an analysis
in blocks of chronological moments in this way has the problem of
reinforcing the notion that periods of time are discrete entities, each with
their own particular characteristics, rather than on-going continuums of
dialectical negotiations with peaks and troughs of activity. Nonetheless, an
analysis based on particular moments is a useful one for a materialist feminist

cultural analysis since it can serve to point out some of the complexities of the relationship between cultural producers, their re-presentations of images, and the audiences/readers who actively consume cultural products. In semiotic terms, this is an attempt to read texts and images synchronically, and then place that reading in a broader diachronic framework. This method enables some conclusions to be drawn about changing meanings in the discourses of femininity, the texts and practices that mediate female identities. Answers were sought to the following questions: why does a particular image of nursing tend to predominate at specific historical conjunctures? How do these images relate to other images of women aimed at female audiences and readers? Which media forms favour the depiction of nurses at certain times and which images gain sufficient critical mass to resonate as remembered influences in personal accounts of nursing identities? Examining these cultural configurations within fictional narratives and recruitment literature reveals how the role of the nurse is given public meaning and status at any given time, and why particular variations of nursing identity predominate in certain periods.

By confining the timescale of this study to the years in which I grew up and became a nurse, I have been able to explore and analyse the socio-cultural contexts of my own subject formation, thereby making personal biography a methodological tool to structure the research and at the same time placing personal experience in a public context. Reading about Florence Nightingale, popularly perceived as the founder of modern nursing, I realised how my own nursing training in the early 1970s had been firmly shaped by her dictates. Like many other schools of nursing, the Liverpool Royal Infirmary was heavily imbued with the Nightingale ethos; its origins lay in the late nineteenth century, when Nightingale's pupil Agnes Jones was instrumental in converting a former eighteenth-century workhouse into a modern institution for housing the sick poor.[8] It became obvious that any attempt to analyse the social relations of my own subject formation as a nurse had to start with more general contexts – such as the legacy bequeathed by images of Nightingale to modern nursing and its professional development.

In the 1980s, feminists became increasingly interested in the role played by popular texts in the formation of female identities. Feminist work on representation has tended to focus either on the psychoanalytic aspects of textual subject formation or on the sociological aspects of social subject formation, often with a difficult correspondence between them. From an initial focus on content analysis, a range of analytical techniques have been developed that tend to emphasise either the formal structure of texts and their unconscious properties (as in much recent feminist film theory) or their reading and interpretative aspects (such as methods of audience ethnography used in media studies). These different approaches, emerging from separate schools of thought, have sometimes had an awkward correspondence.[9] This is partly because the structures of academic disciplines and their institutional frameworks can be a barrier to the creation of fluid inter-disciplinary and multi-disciplinary knowledges. Here, a range of methods drawn from different disciplines are used to argue that the white middle-class images of femininity that represent nursing and nurses in popular fiction and recruitment literature throughout the post-war period were not only representative of professional ideals and practices but also constitutive of those ideals and practices.

This approach to the image is distinctly genealogical; rather than searching for roots or origins it aims to reveal the networks of power relations inscribed in everyday practices.[10] Around the time that I was born, nursing was undergoing fundamental changes as a result of the re-organisation of the health services in Britain into a state-controlled nationalised system. Re-organisation increased the demand for general nurses working in hospitals, and led to new demarcations in nursing work. The play of mediations between the ideals, practices and institutional formations of professional nursing at any one time, dominant ideological notions of femininity, and personal desires and aspirations shapes nursing selves. These conceptual configurations take different forms at different times and in different places but are always, in the final instance, socially, institutionally and individually determined.[11]

The feminist sociologist Dorothy Smith argues that femininity can be read as a collection of texts and discourses that offer a range of choices of how to live life gendered female (1988b). The active engagement with texts that Smith advocates gives female social identity a dynamic, contingent quality which I find in accord with my own experiences – as a shop worker and waitress, nurse and community worker and, more latterly, academic – all of which demand a specific public presentation of the self. Finding out why people make certain choices at particular times, and the influence of popular images on those choices, is an important area for feminists working with popular texts to investigate. Representations of nursing in various forms – stories, pictures, books, films and recruitment literature – are all part of a textually mediated discourse in which individual decisions about becoming a nurse can take place. Smith's theory seems to suggest that there are no limitations to the feminine identities individuals can select, but to bowdlerise a commonly cited expression from Marx, women often make these choices under conditions not of their own choosing. Within this context, nursing becomes potentially available as a choice of job or career for some (but not all) women.[12]

Chapter 1 provides a theoretical framework for the context of the overall analysis. Professional groups generate their own genealogies, often drawing on the names of 'great' leaders or innovators who are identified with the profession's mission as exemplary figures to emulate. Florence Nightingale is an example of such a figure in nursing; her name is enshrined as a national hero in historical records and popular mythology as the founder of the modern profession. For much of the twentieth century her image represented nursing's core ideals and values, her influence pervading both the professional and the public imaginations as one of a few 'good and great' English women. Her writings provide a key to understanding the British context in which images of nurses circulate.

An account of her image is followed by a summary of the commentary on nursing's professional image written exclusively by nurses, most of which emanates from American scholars who focus on content, on the roles performed by nurses in the media and popular fictions. Content analysis contributes a valuable understanding to the ways that female nurses are represented in popular culture; as, for example, ministering angels, doctors' handmaidens, battleaxes and sex objects.[13] The method enables comparisons to be drawn between different textual forms (e.g. TV documentaries and popular romances) and at different times, as well as providing empirical evidence of superficial and unjust media treatment, but it is not the only methodological tool that is useful. Work developed in feminist cultural studies analyses the social relations of image construction. It aims to reveal common assumptions that are constantly reinforced through what Butler (1992) terms reiteration, the process whereby images create a closed circuit of self-reference through constant repetition, reinforcing their iconic status. The reiterated images of nursing that pepper our TV screens are the products of various technologies, institutional organisations and discourses, epistemologies and practices. They are not reproductions of the real conditions of nursing work or symbolic manifestations of those conditions but material practices constructed across a range of sites that interweave and overlap, sometimes conflicting with and contradicting each other.

These practices construct subject positions, imaginary possibilities of how to live as a gendered subject who is also positioned and inscribed by discourses of, amongst others, race, class and age. Subjectivity is the process whereby individuals become subjected to institutional frameworks of regulation and knowledge and produce themselves as subjects. Subject positions are circumscribed by access; as Beverly Skeggs argues, we do not all have equal access to positions in discourse, just as we do not all have equal access to educational opportunities or to the ways in which we can convert our cultural capital into economic capital in the job market (Skeggs 1997: 12). This does not mean that we unquestioningly accept the ways in which we are discursively positioned as subjects; resistance is always an option. Nurses have contested and resisted the ways in which they are constructed and positioned through, for example, protests and campaigns, actions that intervene in the construction of their media identities. One result of these interventions is that some representations hold greater currency at particular historical moments than others. Empirical analysis in the form of case studies and interviews with nurses, the subjects of representation, complements work with media texts to reveal the implicit underlying social relations in representations of nurses and nursing in the post-war period.

Professional critiques of nursing's image have often 'blamed' the media for perpetuating outmoded stereotypes, taking little account of the role the media plays in constructing our notions of what is 'realistic'. Chapter 2 pays particular attention to how the 'realisticness' or 'common sense' of nursing's professional identity is socially constructed by focusing on the depiction of nurses and nursing in images produced across a range of media sites. It examines the social relations that structure the public imaginary, mapping changes in the mediation of professional identity and arguing that the media intervene actively in the social construction of reality as we know and experience it. The ways in which Western media products dominate our TV screens, cinemas, book shops and newspaper stands make it easy to forget that the view-point we are invariably presented with, whether it is looking outwards or reflecting on our own political, cultural and social life, is invariably Anglo-European or American, usually white and most frequently male and middle-class. This has significant implications for nursing as a gendered profession because it compounds what Celia Davies (1995) has identified as the 'professional predicament' in nursing. Davies argues that the attempt to define and shape the nature of nursing work in debates about health care policy frequently results in marginalisation or silencing. Media representations of nurses often reinforce this situation, (re)presenting nurses as the sentimental romantic interest or background presences in the medical dramas enacted around them. On the one hand, nurses are highly valued as individuals but on the other hand, nursing, defined as women's work, is devalued and given low status in society.

The image of an occupational group or profession that is (re)presented in the media is often taken axiomatically as a measure of that group's social and economic value. Nursing's public image has been a source of concern to its leaders for some time. In January 1999 Rachael Thackery in *The Independent* reported that low recruitment was creating a national shortage of nurses with an estimated 13,000 unfilled vacancies nation-wide. The report claimed that the reason why nursing fails to attract sufficient numbers of well-motivated students is a poor public image; the professional response to such critiques has tended to blame the media for reinforcing old-fashioned ideas of what nursing really is all about. In Chapter 3, the recruitment literature produced by the profession and the government in the 1950s, 1960s and 1970s is analysed with these claims very much in mind.

Stories and images of nursing lives, both public and familial, help to shape our nursing subjectivities, our sense of a 'nursing self', our personal sense of who we are, what nursing work entails and how that work is valued. Representations create a cognitive and an emotional framework in which expectations, aspirations and frustrations are given material form and substance. Representations, by their very nature, mediate our experiences of everyday life and are one of the primary means through which we make sense of our selves (or not) and our material realities. Chapter 4 argues that the personal imagination – how nurses construct themselves – is an integral aspect of nursing's occupational identity. The voices recorded here are found in autobiographies and personal narratives of nursing lives; in these accounts, structural formations of gender, class and race are shown to shape the experience of becoming a nurse and, ultimately, the nursing self. In the post-war world the social constraints of gender, class capital and 'race' cannot be separated from how one becomes a nurse, where training is undertaken and the career opportunities available.

The accounts of their nursing lives told by Barbadian women reveal that the white middle-class identity of nursing that dominated popular fictions and recruitment literature throughout this period was not only representative of nursing ideals and practices but also helped shape those ideals and practices. In spite of the enormous changes in patient care brought about by changes in medico-scientific knowledge and the re-organisation of the health services, professional status and autonomy in nursing continued to be anchored to a white, feminine ideal rather than locating itself in the specific skills, methods and knowledge of nursing practice. As the interviewees reveal, their images of what might constitute a 'proper nurse' have – like my own – much in common with the dominant nursing discourses of the time. But their reflections and reconstructions of their nursing lives give voice to some of the disjunctions and ambivalences that have fractured the 'feminine ideal' concealed within the discourse of the 'proper' nurse. By the late 1960s, nurses were publicly questioning and challenging passive models of professional identity, exposing the tensions hidden behind cheerful images of devotion and supplicancy and revealing the colonising assumptions of the professionalisers. Other narratives of nursing history are revealed in these accounts, narratives of assimilation and difference told by experienced practitioners of their struggles to claim value and status for nursing work. These testimonies can be found in the National Sound Archive, where, at the time of writing, they constitute the only unofficial record of nurses' voices talking about their working lives in the post-war period.[14]

Chapter 5 analyses contemporary images of professional identity within the context of equal opportunities discourse. Since the 1970s, laws against discrimination on the grounds of gender and/or race have generated a slow shift in some British institutions towards fairer employment practices;[15] in nursing, as in the National Health Service (NHS) more generally, the pace of change has been uneven (Beishon, Virdee and Hagell 1995). In British media institutions such as broadcasting, the legislation has met a mixed response ranging from the provision of programmes targeted at minority audiences to more inclusive strategies that situate white women and black women and men as presenters of national news. The implications of these changes for nursing's public image are traced in the final chapter which examines contemporary fictions aimed at young people as well as the prevalence of nursing images on terrestrial television.

The research aimed to explore popular formations of a modern image of femininity, the imaginary frameworks that mediated nursing as a social role and a personal identity for women primarily in the post-war period. It has achieved three notable contributions to the development of work in this area: the first is an empirical study of a wide range of material which now provides a unique record of how nursing was popularly represented in Britain at the time; the second is an analysis of nursing's identity focused on issues of gender, class and race that foregrounds assumptions of professional nursing as an identity for young, middle-class white women and those who aspire to such status; and finally, the use of autobiography to frame the timespan of the work places the relationship between images circulating in the popular memory, official accounts of nursing history and newly voiced memories of those events and experiences in a useful genealogical tension that foregrounds the researcher's role in the research process.

Exploring a modern myth of femininity in some detail is an inconclusive activity; it helps us know more about the world we live in or have lived in, rather than breaching new theoretical frontiers or providing statistics to support policies for change. Nonetheless, this kind of cultural work is important and necessary; locating how different images of femininity are defined and organised depends on how more general processes involved in constructing images, meanings and identities are understood, which can lead to very different strategies for resistance or change.

1

IMAGES, IDENTITIES AND SELVES

Every woman, or at least almost every woman in England
has, at one time or another in her life, charge of the personal
health of somebody, whether child or invalid – in other words,
every woman is a nurse.
(Florence Nightingale quoted in Poovey 1989: 185)

Since Nightingale's day, nursing and female identity have been difficult to
prise apart. Often identified as the founder of modern nursing, and the
only woman to appear on a banknote in modern Britain, Nightingale's
image has entered the realms of popular mythology as one of a very few
'good and great' English women. Feminist historians have revealed,
however, that Nightingale's image was mobilised, even in her own time,
to serve colonial and nationalistic aspirations. In her ambition to forge a
profession for women and rally middle-class women to her cause,
Nightingale (re)presented images of the Victorian middle-class mother, the
'angel in the house', as nursing's feminine ideal. But Nightingale also
mobilised another now more hidden discourse that has popularly survived
in the figure of 'the battleaxe'; this military image of authoritarian female
power served an explicitly colonialist aim of reforming and recreating the
home of the sick poor into a facsimile of the female, middle-class home.
In her examination of Nightingale's use of rhetoric, Mary Poovey argues
that the Victorian ideal of submission and domesticity always contained an
aggressive component. For Nightingale, the role of the nurse was not only
to care for the sick, but to become a public agent of moral reform, and
through this agency, ultimately to undermine the power of medical men
(Poovey 1989: 191–2).

The self-sacrificing 'angel' and the 'battleaxe' are not necessarily dia-
metrically opposed. The roots of the 'angel' image arguably lie in the mid-
nineteenth-century promotion of Nightingale as an 'angel of mercy', a
public relations exercise that aimed to pacify public dissatisfaction with the
losses (both military and financial) incurred during the Crimean War
(F. Smith 1982: 47).[1] In the aftermath of her return, Nightingale, a consum-
mate strategist, used her heroic public status to reform nursing, drumming
up support for her projects through an appropriation of the caring

10

characteristics associated with 'respectable', middle-class women circulating in nineteenth-century society (Poovey 1989).

Vron Ware argues that, in Britain, although the concept of femininity has been deconstructed by feminist historians as a class-specific phenomenon, it is rarely investigated to reveal the racial meanings attached to being a white woman (Ware 1992). The first section of this chapter argues that the power value of white femininity, with its cultural associations of chastity, purity, cleanliness and spiritual truth, was used by Nightingale in her attempts to persuade the male-dominated Victorian public sphere to support her programme of reform. Nursing's integral association with the dominant discourse of white middle-class femininity at this time means that it cannot be separated from the racial implications inherent in the reform movements of the day. Nursing was deeply implicated in the colonial and nationalistic ambitions of Victorian society, bequeathing modern nursing an invisible legacy that has permeated the image and identity of professional nursing for much of the twentieth century.[2]

Since the mid-1970s, nursing commentators have become increasingly critical of images of professional identity circulating in the mass media, claiming that nursing is misrepresented and poorly understood by producers, writers and visual image makers. Content analysis, the methodological approach favoured by many researchers of nursing's occupational identity and public image, yields useful and necessary information on how nurses are represented across a range of media sites, but it often fails to reveal the implicit nature of the social relations on which these explicit meanings are fabricated. Analyses of nursing's public image can be usefully developed using the theories and methods of feminist cultural studies, which argues that knowledge is always situated and located in particular schools of thought or epistemes which feminist academics aim to challenge and subvert. Feminist nursing historians and academics can assist this process through their analyses of the public image and identity of nursing as a discourse mediated through conceptions of white middle-class femininity. If this image, with its associative elements of class and colonial subjugation, is to be dislodged from its hegemonic mediation of nursing's occupational identity, differences within nursing and between nurses have to be recognised and treated with respect. It is not only the attitudes of image makers and producers that need to be swayed; there is no place for complacency in nursing's professional associations. In April 1999, in the wake of the controversial judgement of institutional racism within the Metropolitan Police following a public inquiry into the racially motivated murder of Stephen Lawrence, the Royal College of Nursing (RCN) voted against instituting a policy of positive discrimination to tackle racism in the profession.[3] The result generated despair and despondency amongst black nurses and a fierce debate that culminated in a second vote with a more positive outcome.[4] The incident underlines the fact that stereotypes often contain within them implicit truths; nursing's discursive formations will be unable to mediate a fresh identity for the profession until the majority of nurses can envisage a different and more diverse image of their professional selves.[5]

Images: nursing and femininity

The contemporary dilemma faced by nursing historians and feminists in any attempt to account for the gendered identity of health care professionalism is posed acutely in terms of how the image of Florence Nightingale is situated in what Dorothy Smith terms the discourse of femininity (Smith 1988b). Smith argues that femininity can be examined as an actual practice, as a social form of consciousness that takes place in real time, in real places within a defined set of material circumstances. Her focus 'investigates a lived world of on-going social action organised textually' through the production, distribution and consumption of all forms of texts (Smith 1988b: 39). For Smith, femininity is an active enterprise; women construct their feminine identities (or not) through their daily interaction with magazines, books, television and films (to name but a few examples) and the purchase of the products they promote. Textually mediated discourse is a distinctive feature of everyday life in contemporary Western societies that has its roots in the development of mass communications and literacy in the nineteenth century.[6] The consumption and interpretation of texts such as photographs, newspapers, books, magazines and, more recently, radio, film and television are an integral aspect of everyday life. These texts contribute to the organisation of individual choice and the understanding of personal and social experiences as well as mediating the social relations of the political process and the economy (Hermes 1995, Silverstone 1994). Phenomenologists, in their quest to elucidate the relations between experience and knowledge, argue that lived experience consists of interpreted realities; meaning is the relationship established between the self and its everyday experiences.[7] For Smith, women are not passive products of social and economic organisation: they actively create themselves through interactions with their everyday worlds (1988a). In this context, femininity is a set of texts and practices that socialise and teach women how to live our lives as gendered individuals, enabling us to select and reject those aspects of feminine appearance, behaviour and attitudes that suit (or not) our individual needs, attitudes and circumstances. Femininity is a 'textually mediated discourse', a dialectical process between active, creative individuals and the organisation of their behaviour in and through texts that co-ordinate their activities with the market in goods and services. The emphasis here is not on the text itself (as in much conventional literary study) or its content and effects (as in some media and communications sociology and psychology) but on the social relations that are implicated in and through the textual construction of practices.

Smith's analysis of femininity as a practice mediated by the social relations of different kinds of texts is usefully enlarged by Beverly Skeggs, who argues that femininity is a form of cultural capital that women are encouraged to inhabit and practise. The texts and practices of femininity are taken up and used variously by women, whose choices are informed by the network of social relations they inhabit. Positions of class, gender, sexuality, race, religion, region and age, for example, ensure that the discourses of femininity are taken up (and resisted) in different ways. Skeggs' longitudinal study of a group of young women who returned to further education to study courses in community care demonstrates how the group were encouraged to convert their everyday skills (of caring for children and tending to the needs of others) into marketable skills. Femininity is a form of cultural capital that can be transformed into economic capital but it is a limited resource in that it only provides restricted access to potential forms of power, whereas it is possible to trade masculinity more readily and for greater reward in the labour market (Skeggs 1997: 10).

Textually mediated discourse does more than communicate popular sentiments and values: it connects the production and distribution of, for example, clothes, furnishings, and education with the skills and work (paid and unpaid) of women, and the norms and images that both construct and regulate the public presentation of the self in the social realm. Within the discourse of femininity, women are situated as objects not only of a male desiring gaze, but also of their own self-disciplining gaze. Smith describes the structure of the relationship of the subject to herself as tripartite: 'the distance between herself as a subject and her body, which becomes the object of her work, is created by the textual image through which she becomes conscious of its defects' (Smith 1988b: 50). This relationship is often foregrounded in accounts of anorexia which Chenin (1983, quoted in Smith) has suggested is a conflict in which some women cannot resolve the relations between mind and body. Smith sees this conflict as an over-intensification of an already existing tension between the subject, textual images and the 'body-as-object-of-work'; participation in the discourse of femininity situates the body as an object of the work involved in trying to achieve the unchanging perfection of the image in the text. Thus Toni Morrison's heroine Pecola in her novel *The Bluest Eye* (1970) sees herself as black and ugly, her body as the object of work involved in trying to achieve the textually mediated norm of white feminine beauty. Unable to create a transformation through the consumption of products aimed at young white women, she seeks a magical solution from a black soothsayer that will make her dream come true. Finally, she goes mad because she cannot make her body conform to the idealised images of white femininity that are consuming her sense of self – in the magazines, advertisements and movies that surround her (Smith 1988b).

Poovey (1984) has mapped the genealogy of femininity's discursive development, tracing its emergence to the eighteenth-century production of magazines and conduct books addressed to leisured upper-class women. This situates femininity as a class discourse, one that places women in a social hierarchy in which economic wealth and social relations are productive of certain forms of female conduct and appearance. In the nineteenth century, books and articles in magazines as well as advertisements created a common code among readers, vested in languages and images which could be referenced in conversation and in interpreting behaviour and events. Conduct books provided instruction on how to become a 'lady' for growing numbers of socially aspirant women, the wives and daughters of (newly) wealthy entrepreneurs, industrialists, merchants and emerging professionals eager to join upper- and upper middle-class society. The development of textual and visual technologies, such as printing and photography, emphasised the construction of appearance as a sign of female conduct that implied social respectability. By the end of the century, appearance became a signifier of conduct with hair styles and clothes the predominant means through which middle-class women could define themselves and place others. Femininity was established as a certain kind of womanhood, a middle-classed sign that connoted the particular forms of conduct deemed 'respectable'. Investments in the social trappings of this idealised form of femininity enabled women to gain access to limited status and moral superiority. Donning the accoutrements of their social positioning and displaying them through appearance enabled white middle-class women to judge those who were lacking in 'femininity' (feminine class capital) as inferior. Hence 'respectability' became not only an indication of social status but also of moral value and social worth (Skeggs 1997: 100–1).

Skeggs argues that white middle-class femininity was defined as the ideal but also as the most passive and dependent of femininities. Working-class women were paradoxically coded: on the one hand, they were depicted as inherently healthy, hardy and robust in contrast to the frail physical bodies and 'delicate' temperaments of middle-class women; on the other hand, they were seen as a source of infection and disease, in part the result of their 'dangerous' sexual appetites. Working-class women's relationship to femininity has historically been predicated on a class-based relationship to the vulgar, the pathological and the sexual; they are distanced from 'taste', from the static, silent, invisible and composed forms of conduct and behaviour which are the marks of respectability (Davidoff 1983, Stanley 1984, Skeggs 1997).

Women and caring have strong cultural associations in Western culture, which can lead to assumptions that caring is a natural or essential attribute of those born female, a genetic inheritance rather than a socially learnt pattern of behaviour. But many feminists have challenged the supposition that females are 'naturally' more caring than males, arguing that caring is a socially acquired attribute, part of the process of gendering female identity in Western cultures through the discourse of femininity.[8] An important

14

theme of early nineteenth-century women's history is the philanthropic, caring role often assigned to women of the emerging middle classes. Nightingale's relationship to the Victorian feminist movement has been a source of considerable interest and debate amongst feminist nursing scholars and historians: her association with Victorian philanthropic movements and British imperial power is well documented although it has not been subjected to a sustained critique of its racial implications.[9] Feminine discourse ascribed special qualities of a moral and ethical nature to middle-class women which defined the domestic realm as their principal area of responsibility and operation. This is sometimes referred to as 'woman's mission': women were expected to use their special qualities as a reforming influence on family and friends and to donate their leisure time and energy to societies engaged in social and moral reform.

One of the contradictions of 'woman's mission' is that it helped to regulate the distance between women of different social classes. Linda Nead discusses the way the phrase was used to describe the role of the respectable woman in the reclamation of 'the fallen' (prostitutes and other women of dubious morality), and the way that it differentiated between the 'deserving' and 'undeserving' poor (Nead 1988: 196–7). Philanthropic work also constructed hierarchical relationships between white women and those of different races. Vron Ware argues that it was a short step from bestowing charity on poor women to applying the same principles of compassion to assist and plead for those who were enslaved, a more abstract group of poor with whom white middle-class women had little physical contact.[10] The urban poor belonged to a social hierarchy that was familiar to middle-class women; their condition could be addressed by Bible readings or education in home economics, but not by campaigning for their emancipation or their equality. The abolition of slavery was a political struggle aimed at changing hearts, minds and laws; it could be read as merely sentimental philanthropy but it could also signify an assault on racism itself (Ware 1992). The abolitionist movement allowed women to use their image of respectability in the public sphere, but the success of the campaign was followed, paradoxically, by an increase in British imperial control of many areas of the world. The relationship between white women and those of different races continued to evolve during the nineteenth century through their participation in the British colonising project (Ware 1992: 109); missionary work, nursing, teaching and marriage to colonial officials expanded the reach of 'woman's mission' way beyond their own 'urban jungles'.[11] Wendy Webster points out that the analogy between British colonial and urban English missionary work was often made explicit; William Booth, founder of the Salvation Army, described the urban poor as 'colonies of heathen savages in the heart of our capital', arguing that: 'As there is a darkest Africa is there not also a darkest England?'[12] (quoted in Webster 1998: 62).

The 1850s were something of a watershed in women's history, for it was in this decade that discursive formations of femininity became distinctly allied to various reform movements, creating discrete and separate identities for groups of middle-class women that were predicated on their religious and political attitudes and beliefs. Nightingale's reforming mission, which culminated in the opening of her School of Nursing, is perhaps the most well-known and publicly acclaimed activity of this type during the decade, but her projects were accompanied by two other significant interventions. In 1858 one of the first feminist publications, *The Englishwoman's Journal*, started publishing with the explicit aims of generating support for the opening up of skilled occupations to women and of raising the status of acceptable female occupations such as nursing and teaching (Simnett 1986). In the following year, 1859, the Ladies Association for the Diffusion of Sanitary Knowledge (LADSK) was founded by evangelical middle-class women who saw it as their moral duty to visit the poor and teach them about the virtues of fresh air, good diet, clean clothes and houses and clean living. These middle- and upper-class women, in a manner that forecasts the development of the Health Visiting movement some fifty years later, visited the houses of the poor in an attempt to redeem working-class women from themselves, that is from themselves as a sign of dangerous, disruptive sexual women (Hall 1979 in Skeggs 1997: 99). At the inaugural ceremony of LADSK the celebrated novelist Charles Kingsley urged women to recognise that 'one of the noblest duties' was 'to help the increase of the English race as much as possible' in order to colonise the Empire (Ware 1992: 247, quotations in original). By the 1870s the charitable work of white middle-class evangelical woman was still aimed at educating her working-class counterpart in religion, morality and sanitation. As the ideology of Empire developed, the sphere of influence of white middle-class evangelical women expanded to the colonial territories captured and dominated by the British; personal cleanliness had become not only an index of class difference, but it also provided the measure of civilisation in other countries. Gender played a crucial role in organising ideas of 'race' and 'civilisation'; women were involved in many different ways in the expansion and maintenance of the Empire. Hammerton argues that 'notions of imperial destiny and class and racial superiority were grafted onto the traditional views of refined English motherhood to produce a concept of the Englishwoman as an invincible global civilising agent' (A. J. Hammerton, *Emigrant Gentlewoman*, in Mackay and Thane 1986: 28–9). The presence of white women demanded, for example, that relations between the 'races' be highly regulated. The increasing number of white women who travelled out to join husbands and families in the colonies, or to work in their own right as missionaries, nurses and teachers, often had far-reaching effects on the social lives of white male settlers, and consequently on the status and sexual exploitation of black women (Ware 1992: 38).

The popular assertion that 'cleanliness is next to godliness', while it reveals fears of moral pollution and physical contagion from sexual licentiousness and diseases associated with the poverty of overcrowded urban slums, hides an underlying discourse of racial hygiene. Richard Dyer argues that the power value of whiteness resides in its apparent neutrality; but the colour white carries an explicit symbolic sense of moral and aesthetic superiority with an emphasis on purity, spirituality, truth, cleanliness and chastity. Nineteenth-century racialist thought intertwined science, religion and aesthetics, 'defining Aryans or Caucasians as the pinnacle of the human race in every respect', including physical beauty (Dyer 1997: 71). Non-white peoples were associated with dirt, with bodily emissions and body odours considered distasteful to the 'civilised' sensibilities of white Victorians.[13] White masculinist science and epistemology is constructed around conceptual frameworks of binary classification that place 'man' in a position of dominance over the natural world: mind is superior to body, culture to nature, reason to emotion, knowing to being, self to others, objectivity to subjectivity. In each pair, Sandra Harding argues, the former is set to control the latter, lest the latter overwhelms the former: in social hierarchies of masculine dominance the threatening 'latter' in each case appears to be associated with the feminine; in the case of racial dominance it is associated with non-Europeans (Harding, quoted in Ware 1992: 37).

Gender and race do not sit neatly on one or other side of this binary system of conceptual classification; civilisation is positioned oppositionally to savagery, but in the context of nineteenth-century scientific thought, white women are constructed as essentially uncivilised and primitive, ruled by instinct rather than rationality because of the small size of their brains. Patriarchal thought conceptualises woman as 'the other'; she is associated with nature, the body and the 'pollution' of menstruation; women are the unknowable 'dark continent', lacking reason and self-control, ruled by their wombs rather than their heads.[14] In the context of imperialism, patriarchal ideology places white women firmly in the civilised camp in opposition to non-European women whose colour and lack of social, economic and political rights is regarded by white colonisers as a sign of cultural savagery (Ware 1992: 237). Thus white women can occupy both sides of the dichotomous formulations of Western thought and the social relations that they inscribe and organise. Nursing cannot extricate itself from this web of historical associations; as a caring occupation gendered female it is situated in an inferior relationship to the scientific project of bio-medicine, but the professionalising project of nursing supports the colonising projects of British imperialism.[15] In her examination of Nightingale's use of rhetoric, Mary Poovey argues that the two fronts on which Nightingale waged her war for nursing supremacy had their counterparts in the two fronts on which England's middle-class men waged their war for cultural and economic supremacy. The two discourses employed 'the same terms in different social registers: the patient (read: India, the poor) is really a brute (a native, a working-class man) who must be cured (colonised, civilised) by an efficient head nurse cum bourgeois mother (England, middle-class women)'. The ultimate goal, in both cases, is to transform society through surveillance, discipline, and good administration presided over by a 'house-wifely, regal, classless woman' (1989: 196). This woman is, in the first instance, Queen Victoria, the 'mother' of the nation, and in the second, Nightingale's vision of the reformed nurse, the 'mother' who cares for the sick individual.[16]

Deconstructing her popular image, Poovey points out that Nightingale used a diverse range of strategies in her writings in order to secure a broad spectrum of public support for her innovative schemes. This has enabled her 'to be read', both in her own time and subsequently, as a supporter of various reform movements that are quite at odds with each other ideo-logically, such as the suffragette movement and the Victorian cult of true womanhood. Pointing out how Nightingale's representation of nursing was in fact her greatest success, Poovey argues that Nightingale was a good tactical strategist who used written discourse to achieve her aims and ambi-tions. Her symbolic reworking of the image of the nurse at mid-century was complex: in order to attract young, middle-class women, nursing had to be freed from the taint of its lower-class origins but also from the spectre of the 'strong minded women' who wanted to be doctors. These two images were part of the social construct of the image of the nurse embraced by the public. Sairey Gamp, the infamous drunken nurse created by Dickens in *Martin Chuzzlewit*, galvanised the prejudices and anxieties of a large sector of the English public. Despite occasional acknowledgements that good nurses did exist before Nightingale, many commentators of the day reviled nurses for their bad temper and drunkenness, representing them as irresponsible fools only interested in money. Reformers used the same tactic: according to Nightingale, 'Nurses were women who were too old, too weak, too drunken, too dirty, too stolid, or too bad to do anything else' (quoted in Poovey 1989: 174).

Nightingale's public reputation secured her a dominant ideological posi-tion in the reform of nursing: by combining nineteenth-century feminine values with modern ideas about the organisation of hospital work, she created the conditions that enabled women to join her in the fight against dirt and moral corruption that was the lynchpin of her mission. In its day, this was an exciting and attractive alternative to the medical model of health care, one that contained the promise of empowering women through nursing. Martha Vicinus points out that in the first 'pioneer' stage of nursing reform (1850s–1880s), Nightingale and her followers recruited and trained the kinds of women who saw themselves as soldiers in the fight against disease, serving a cause that was organised hierarchically according to a military model. Recruits were drawn from middle-class families with sufficient money to educate their daughters (such as the clergy) but not enough to support them should they never marry. Class snobbery was an explicit part of the recruitment process and was successful because few other vocations, even those of headmistress or mother superior, 'offered such a grand opportunity for effecting visible change in a male-dominated world' (Vicinus 1985: 95). This hierarchical system of control and its underlying military ideology were reinforced for the second generation of recruits through the use of maternal metaphors which strengthened the control of nursing's upper middle-class reforming leaders. In both periods, it was class superiority that gave women the confidence to drive through the nursing reforms, but by the end of the century, this female vision could not survive the growing power of bio-medicine and the consolidation of medical control of all aspects of health care provision. Nurses could only maintain their power and respect by exaggerating the differences between the treatment given by doctors and the care administered by nurses; nursing leaders argued for a distinct, separate and unequal place for women which was subordinate to medicine but controlled by themselves (Vicinus 1985, Gamarnikow 1991).

Dorothy Smith (1988b) argues that the distinctive property of textually mediated discourse is its capacity to organise local practices and relationships in multiple sites. Nursing, like femininity, is not a unitary construct; in the struggles between different interest groups for control of the profession, general hospital nursing has gained prominence, its image dominating that of other nursing identities such as psychiatric, geriatric and community nursing. In the nineteenth century, most (non-private household) nursing took place in an assortment of institutions ranging across high profile, voluntary hospitals run by subscription and charitable donations, large municipal fever and psychiatric institutions funded from local rates, and small rural infirmaries with a tradition of care based on the administration of the Poor Law. Within these different organisations, nursing recruitment and training were unevenly organised: on one level, the high status London charity hospitals attracted educated, middle-class young women, some with ambitious career horizons. In less privileged institutions, the workforce was considerably more diverse and, in the case of Poor Law institutions, nursing was often undertaken by widows who were forced to earn a living because of their reduced circumstances. This range of services, with their own local, regional and national variations, created uneven patterns of recruitment and training. Ann Simnett argues that by the beginning of the twentieth century, nursing was not the solid middle-class occupation that a study of the London hospitals alone might suggest. Increasing opportunities in an expanding area of work that had acquired a respectable reputation drew young white women, often from lower middle-class backgrounds, into the training schools (Simnett 1986).

The mythologisation of Nightingale, both in her own time and subsequently, has led to her image sustaining what are now seen as apparently conflicting images of nursing. Nightingale is known as the self-sacrificing angel, the 'lady with the lamp', as well as an efficient administrator and leader. She is both the tender, compassionate, bedside nurse dedicated to the physical and psychological welfare of her patient, and 'the battleaxe', the tough, determined head nurse who creates order out of chaos and runs her unit with military efficiency. Public formations of nursing's professional identity are inseparable from the constructs of femininity that give them substance and meaning at any one time. I will argue that in the post-war period, the public images of the nurse – the white angel, the doctor's handmaiden, the battleaxe and the sexy nurse – shift in relation to nursing's internal structural relations of gender, race and class as well as in relation to changing notions of women's role in society. Many commentators have argued that these stereotypical images misrepresent nursing and it is to that critique that I will now turn my attention.

Identities: nurses and their professional image

Nursing's relationship to femininity is a recurring theme in much of the literature on images of nursing that has emanated from the profession. What most of this literature has in common is a concern with the content of popular fictional forms, and how nurses are represented in them. The binary stereotypes of femininity, the virgin and the whore, take on a set of particular characteristics in nursing images that have their origins in early nineteenth-century ideas about the 'essential' nature of the feminine. The 'good' nurse is invariably seen as a form of self-sacrificing angel who gives up everything to dedicate her life to caring for the sick; the 'bad' nurse is her exact opposite, misusing her position of power and authority to satisfy her own needs and desires, whether these are material, sexual or simply sadistic. While these images can always be closely mapped against other prevailing images of women at any one time, the argument presented in this book is that nursing policy and practice adapts or resists these more general currents in various ways at particular times.

A considerable body of writing now addresses these polarised figurations of nursing femininity. Feminist critiques of the representation of women in popular culture in the 1970s and 1980s argue that these images are constructed by male-dominated economic institutions that construct and project male fantasies of women.[17] The sign 'Woman' cannot adequately address the real relations of women in society; it is an imaginary signifier, a product of a patriarchal unconsciousness that has no roots in the re-presentation of the real conditions of existence.[18] Representational systems function on the continual reproduction of the sign 'Woman', reinforcing their signifying power through constant repetition and self-reference, creating an imaginary framework of representation of the 'real' world that is ideologically implicated in power relations. The constant reiteration of stereotypes reinforces dominant conceptions of 'Woman'; attitudinal behaviours such as self-sacrifice, obedience, loyalty and devotion are given high moral and ethical value and are represented as normative behaviour for 'good' women. Qualities such as self-determination, assertiveness and leadership are given negative connotations when attached to females (the 'battleaxe' syndrome), but in males are highly valued. Regimes of representation function on these dichotomous conceptual categories of difference, their polarisations both reflecting and constructing attitudes and behaviours towards social relations that are distinguished by, amongst other distinctions, differences of gender, class and race.

Post-1970s critiques of nursing's image adapt this conceptual framework of analysis, adopting an approach which tends to 'blame' the mass media for promoting false myths and fantasies. Nurses began to challenge media stereotypes, claiming that misrepresentation was leading to a poorly understood perception of their role by the public. In 'Will the "real" nurse please stand up: the stereotype versus reality', American nurses Elms and Moorehead try to present an alternative vision to dominant fictional representations, claiming that the explaining, analysing and blaming of the image by sociologists, psychologists and feminists respectively is doing little to alter the status quo. Instead they offer 'profiles, descriptions and clarifications to expose and dispel the stereotypes' (Elms and Moorehead 1977: 127).

Following a government inquiry into the image of nursing chaired by the broadcasting historian Asa Briggs (1972), a similar concern with misrepresentation was beginning to be voiced in British nursing circles. In an address to the International Council of Nursing's 16th Quadrennial Congress in Tokyo, Christine Chapman, Director of Advanced Nursing Studies at the National School of Medicine, Wales, presented a paper on the image of the nurse for a special interest session called 'How do we see ourselves and how do others see us?' (Chapman 1977). Chapman claims that in the Western world, the mass media give clues to the images a group of workers may present. Whilst she appreciates the media's need to use stereotypes, she questions the fact that on television nurses are portrayed as female, white, single and dedicated – as 'angels of mercy'. Tracing the history of the nursing image through Dickens' caricature of the pre-Nightingale nurse and the Nightingale reforms, Chapman claims that a positive image of the nurse still exists in the West. She uses recent research conducted by the RCN to prove her point, where it was found that 76 per cent of patients had a positive image and high expectation of nurses, anticipating technical competence accompanied by gentleness, kindness, patience and sympathy (Anderson 1973). She discusses the different expectations of patients, doctors, neophytes, and the profession wanting autonomy and recognition. Chapman asks, 'Can the nurse be all things to all men? Are these images and expectations mutually exclusive?' As a positive step to resolving some of these difficulties, she suggests that the profession can construct a more realistic image of nursing by seeking nurse advisers on TV programmes, correcting statements in the press and learned journals and making recruitment literature more realistic.

In Britain in the early 1980s many of the debates about the representation of nursing tended to be carried out in academic departments focused on questioning and re-writing nursing history (Dingwall and McIntosh 1978, Davies 1980, Maggs 1983 and 1984). In North America, perhaps because of a greater emphasis on degree-level education for nurses, nurses were producing interesting cultural work that foregrounded the question of public opinion through historical studies of popular magazines, novels and newspapers. Hughes' (1980) study 'The public image of the nurse' is typical of this approach, which uses content analysis to formulate generalisations about public opinion and identify themes that emerged in magazines throughout the period 1896–1976. Her concern is motivated by economic considerations: in the privatised USA health care system, the value of nursing work is decided by those who control the budgets. According to Hughes, the mass media have created a mythological image of the ideal nurse; the personality and appearance of the nurse are emphasised, negating the intellectual and educational requirements of nursing practice. Physical fitness was given precedence over intelligence in recruitment drives as late as 1943, and the timbre of the voice was seen as an important attribute. A 1955 edition of *Look* defined the function of the nurse as 'giving injections, back rubs and bed baths [and] making a neat hospital bed'. A 1956 article in *The Reader's Digest* claimed that 'the responsiveness of a nurse comes more from her personality than from her formal education', even though the nurse is required to 'perform delicate tasks and exercise the kind of judgement that until recent years were the exclusive prerogatives of doctors'. As recently as 1971, *Life* reported that as a student nurse, one 'learns the right way to take a blood pressure, read a thermometer – and even empty a bedpan' (Hughes 1980: 63). In addition to these physical typologies and personality traits, Hughes identifies persistent themes running through North American popular literature which are also prevalent in Britain.[19] These can be summarised as nursing as women's work, as 'unwholesome', as virtue personified and as a vocation. Symbolic themes associated with the profession are those of 'the born nurse', 'the new road to matrimony' and 'physician's helpmate'. Interestingly, Hughes does not comment on images that emphasise the sexuality of nurses and their sexual availability, a common theme in American films following the relaxation of censorship in the late 1950s. She argues that nurses will only become established as independent practitioners in their own right once they are paid directly for their services, rather than employed by others to perform those services on their behalf. As the consumers of health care provided by nurses, only the public can create the demand for nursing labour that will ensure nurses function in non-traditional roles in the future.[20]

In a similar vein, Janet Muff's edited collection *Socialisation, Sexism and Stereotyping: Women's Issues in Nursing* (1982) traces the relationship between nursing, gender and femininity from early childhood, through career choice and into professional nursing; a significant collection of essays discuss strategies for change through political action. For these writers, empowering nurses professionally involves situating the self outside the discourses of femininity that continue to pervade professional nursing practice. In the same year, the American Academy of Nursing vowed to develop an action plan that would present nursing as 'the complex, diverse, challenging, brainy, caring profession that it is' (*American Nurse* 1982).

Within the British context, Jane Salvage (1982) was also concerned about myths of nursing perpetuated by media stereotypes. Salvage was the first nurse to write in depth about the range of images in popular circulation in Britain, and how they affect the expectations of those entering the profession, as well as the general public.[21] In 'Angles, not angels', for example, she compares the assertive militancy of nurses during a dispute with their NHS employers with the mass-produced fantasies of Mills & Boon doctor/nurse romances, claiming that these are 'only the most conspicuous of forms that represent nurses as doctors' doting handmaidens', an image that pervades even the NHS recruitment literature (Salvage 1982: 12–13). Salvage is critical of professional collusion in perpetuating outmoded stereotypes, citing a uniform design competition in the *Nursing Times* as an example. The winning entry was an ultra-feminine dress that incorporated many traditional stereotypical features including black stockings, a frilly cap and a white apron, an image rife with connotations of eroticism, vocational duty and housework. Such images reinforce outdated ideas of medical domination and outdated working relationships, and fail to point out the skills and difficulties of nursing work. These myths, she argues, can only be defused by adopting a plurality of images, since any single image is bound to be a crude reduction. 'Nurses must resist cliches, contest the traditional myths and make the fight against sexism a central activity in nursing politics' (Salvage 1982: 13).

Salvage is one of the most forceful advocates of this view on the British nursing scene and has written at length about the relationship between nursing, gender and sexuality (Salvage 1983a, 1985, 1987a, 1987b), but like many analysts who seek to shift the gendered relations in health care, issues of class and race, if they feature, are often treated as an effect of gender inequality, not as a constituent element of that inequality. Salvage claims that black nurses suffer additionally from the way in which the sexuality of black women has become stereotyped (1987a), but this ignores the structural relations of race within nursing itself and the ways in which white middle-class colonial nurses accepted and perpetuated discrimination through hierarchical organisational structures (Marks 1997).[22]

Critiques of gender and sexuality have dominated debates on the image of nursing because of its relationship to the patriarchal structure of medicine, tending to leave other aspects of nursing's ideological formation, such as class and race, comparatively unexamined.[23] While class and race are not the only vectors of difference that come into play in attempts to deconstruct nursing stereotypes, they are foregrounded here because of their influence on labour relations within nursing itself. Nursing is a hierarchical structure in which cultural and educational capital affect the career opportunities of those entering the profession. The ideology of the professionalising group in the post-war period promoted and projected a tenacious cluster of white middle-class attitudes, values and beliefs that motivated exclusion of those who did not meet their ideal of 'respectable' femininity.

The acute problems of recruitment following the inception of the NHS focused much of the analysis of nursing's public image during the late 1940s, 1950s and 1960s on the attitudes of young women towards nursing as a career. This work has a functionalist emphasis: in line with the prevailing academic fashion of the day, it sought cause and effect relationships focused on the problem of identifying the right sort of girls who would be suitable for nursing. MacGuire reviewed and summarised these findings in 1969; her conclusions, drawn from all the empirically researched sources of information available at that time, provide an overview of how 'the public' viewed nursing throughout this period. Interestingly, she points out that in the National Opinion Poll study *Attitudes to Nurses* (1966)[24] nursing was rated higher by women, older people, those in the lower social classes, those who had left school early and those in the Midland and West regions. It was generally considered to require less intelligence than teaching, and most agreed that to be a nurse you had to have a vocation. A large percentage of the sample thought nurses spent a lot of time doing chores, that nurses were subjected to more discipline than was necessary and worked longer hours than most people (MacGuire 1969: 150).

MacGuire claims that for those who have chosen to be nurses and survive the training, 'personal identity is inextricably bound up with identity as a nurse' (1969: 107). What MacGuire fails to point out, which was taken for granted at the time, is that it was *female* identity and nursing identity that were inextricably connected – and in particular, the identities of young, white, upwardly mobile working- and lower middle-class women. For these groups of women, becoming a nurse meant an investment of time and energy in the training process on the basis that they would achieve respectable social status and a career with good prospects; it also entailed an emotional and ethical investment in the moral framework of caring on which the training was based.

Several points can be drawn from this that have particular relevance for the study of popular images of the period. First of all, career choices for women, even by the late 1960s, were extremely limited; perhaps this is one of the reasons why middle-class respondents were more likely to encourage their daughters to nurse than respondents in the lower status income categories, where more than 80 per cent of the substantial sample thought it was difficult to become a nurse. Nonetheless, views about the lower intelligence of nurses, doing chores, the discipline and poor pay, point to middle-class beliefs about the suitability of particular forms of work for women. Secondly, male respondents in general rated nursing less highly than women, preferring their daughters to embark on careers as secretaries or teachers.[25] Thirdly, women of all social classes rated nursing higher than men partly as a result of the limited horizons available to them, but also, perhaps, because of two fascinations which seem to have pervaded many women's fantasies in the post-war world. One of these was with medicine and medical science, manifest in the consumption of all forms of medical programming on television and the prevalence of popular medical romantic fiction. The other, born of an increase in educational opportunity and the relative affluence of post-war society, was with middle-class lifestyles.[26]

MacGuire's overview stands as an interesting benchmark between the functionalist, empirical work on public attitudes that depends on quantitative analysis as a methodological tool, and a trend towards content analysis and issues of representation that follows in the nursing literature of the 1970s and 1980s. Whereas in the earlier period, professional and governmental concerns with the public image of nursing were motivated by the need to find ways of reaching and attracting candidates who could be identified in some way as 'suitable for nursing', in the era following the Briggs Report (1972) the focus shifts to an awareness of how public images misrepresent nurses and the nursing profession.

The 'reality' constructed by the media suits a particular vision of the world, sustaining beliefs in particular ideas and institutions and the power relations they inscribe. Imaginary constructions have social implications: they are not 'only' fictions or, in the case of news and documentary accounts, value-free representations of the material world; they mediate dominant ideas and values, creating insecurity, doubt, and even fear for those excluded from their terms of address. In the post-war world, images of nursing are unrelentingly white and middle-class; for those working in the elite sectors of general nursing such as former voluntary hospitals, this may have seemed to be the apparent 'reality' of nursing at that time. There were no black nurses and few enrolled nurses on the wards of many provincial teaching hospitals in the early 1970s because, as one nursing manager responsible for recruitment put it, 'nursing managers resisted having too many black faces on the wards'.[27] For those arriving in Britain to train as nurses from overseas, the 'reality' inscribed in nursing's public image was rather different; not only were black nurses expected to conform in both appearance and conduct to nursing's white middle-class ideal, they also had to contend with racial discrimination and verbal and physical harassment from patients and colleagues. Amongst those who gave oral testimony to Wendy Webster for her analysis of images of home in post-war Britain and their significance in constructions of gender, race and nation is Elsie George who was recruited in Nigeria to work in nursing in Britain. She recalls a conversation between herself and a colleague, a Welsh woman:

> 'Nurse G, Nurse G' she said.
> I said, 'Yes, Nurse N.'
> 'Did you live in the jungle?'
> I looked and I said, 'Oh yes, Nurse N.'
> 'Nurse G, Nurse G' she said.
> I said 'Yes, Nurse N.'
> 'Were you living at the top of the tree?'
> I said, 'Yes, Nurse N.'
> 'Nurse G, Nurse G. Have you got a tail?'
> 'Yes, Nurse N.'
> 'Were you wearing a grass skirt?'
> I said, 'Yes, Nurse N.' And believe me, I was really upset.
>
> (Quoted from Webster 1998: 103)

Elsie George challenged this construction of herself by inviting Nurse N to look at her 'tail'; following Nurse N's refusal, she produced a photograph of the school children at the Catholic school where she taught. For women from Africa and the Caribbean who came to Britain to train and work as nurses, the images of nursing in all forms of public communication reflected and constructed nursing as an identity for young white women. In this sense, the images were representative of attitudes and values not only of individual nurses, as this account reveals, but of the professional ideals and values that permeated nursing's institutional structures at this time.

Selves: personal conceptions of professional identity

Several of the studies collected by MacGuire (1969) point out that the image of nursing held by a girl was the most important factor in her self-assessed suitability for training,[28] but there is no suggestion of what image that might have been, or evidence of how girls conceived of nurses and nursing during this period. The issue of self-conception and views on professional identity held by nurses themselves are explored in two ways in this research in order to examine popular constructions of self-representation and throw some light onto the question of why some women chose nursing as a job or a career in the post-war period. This two-pronged approach relies on written narratives in the form of autobiographical novels written during the post-war period and its aftermath, and on oral testimonies prompted from memory in the form of case study interviews. Both forms have methodological problems, discussed in more detail below; used together these shortcomings become complementary since they highlight the theoretical problems inherent in any attempt to use forms of narrative as the basis for knowledge about lived experience.

Feminist scholarship has made the relationship between lived experience and knowledge one of its primary concerns. Getting to know about other women's lives and trying to find ways to re-present those lives within official discourses and debates is a major feminist political task. Interesting parallels can be drawn between the struggles of feminist scholars and their desire to legitimate women as subjects of their own discourses, and nurses who have struggled to make nursing an autonomous profession. Both have sought to authenticate their status through intellectual validation and academic credibility, the former through forging Women's Studies as an autonomous discipline in the academy, the latter through applying medico- and socio-scientific criteria to nursing practice. Both have increasingly relied on theory to support their practice and, as a result, both run the risk in their teaching and professional strategies of perpetuating hierarchical divisions and differences between women.[29]

Nurses have rarely been credited with the authorial ability to write about and represent themselves, but many popular romantic novels featuring nurses are written by women who trained as nurses. Nurses have generated a large body of writing that deals with professional issues, primarily in the form of textbooks and histories of nursing and, increasingly since training moved from schools of nursing attached to hospitals into the university system, in the form of research monographs and articles. Traditionally, nursing was seen as both a science and an art, and this was heralded as a strength of the profession. In more recent years, professional nursing has tended to adopt theoretical approaches to care based on abstract models. According to some critics, these models have tended to generate a deficient view of nursing practice that only allows the gaps to show (Benner and Tanner 1987, Benner and Wrubel 1988, Lawler 1991). Stories, narratives and case studies are increasingly seen as a way of understanding nursing practice because they highlight the relationship between theory and practice and open up the thinking and beliefs that underscore much of nursing work. An approach to theory that is grounded in the discourse of practice can be seen as a re-valuation of what it means to practise the art of nursing, giving precedence to skilled practitioners and their experiences rather than abstract ideas and concepts.[30] To quote Derbyshire, who is pioneering this approach in the British context, 'We have a rich vocabulary which describes our deficiencies and our shortcomings, yet we have scarcely begun to develop a meaningful dialogue which reveals nurses' creativity and expertise in caring' (1991: 27). Stories and case studies written by nurses are increasingly used to create that meaningful dialogue.[31]

In terms of feminist scholarship, stories, narratives and case studies are often used to challenge official discourses and interpretations of women's lives. These methods of study, as the Personal Narratives Group point out, are especially useful for illuminating several aspects of gender relations: 'the construction of gendered self-identity; the relationship between the individual and society in the creation and perpetuation of gender norms; and the dynamics of power relations between women and men' (Personal Narratives Group 1989: 5). I would add that these narratives can also illustrate and illuminate our understandings of power relationships between women, particularly those structured by differences of race and class. Because they attempt to place the lived experiences of women within discrete theoretical models rather than trying to settle more universalising arguments about the location of the self, the methods adopted by the Personal Narratives Group are particularly useful in shaping a methodological approach to examining nursing selves. The association between the socially constructed gendered identity of professional nursing and the shaping of this role as a social and personal identity by individual women who become nurses is explored here through written and verbal reconstructions of the processes of becoming a nurse.[32] These accounts reveal how individuals negotiate the discursive gap between social perceptions of the nursing self and personal conceptions of nursing identity.

Framing the self

Writing an account of one's own life can take several forms, of which diaries, memoirs and autobiographies are the most well-known. Each of these forms frames experience in a set of generic conventions, recognisable to writer and reader as a way of conveying personal experience (Heilbrun 1989). Memoirs, for example, tend to be recollections of past events written in the present and therefore have a tendency to be episodic, highlighting events considered by the writer to be of particular importance. Diaries are usually an attempt to faithfully record impressions and events as they occur at the time. Autobiographies can use a mixture of both forms since what is constructed is a narrative, a story of a life.

Feminist scholarship, with its avowed commitment to the relationship between the personal and the political, has found in women's autobiographical writing a form which seems ideologically appropriate to feminism.[33] Lury (1991) considers that the use of the first person pronoun in autobiographical writing can be seen as indicative of subjective awareness, implying a degree of political self-consciousness at least as far as it claims an authorial right to speak of personal experience. However, the notion of authenticity of autobiographical writing has received extensive criticism from within feminism as well as from without on the grounds that although the heroine (*sic*) is presented as a self-speaking subject, the writer remains tied to traditional forms and values such as the use of linear narrative and an emphasis on female sexuality as the key to women's identity. This raises problems for a feminist analysis because of an underlying implication that biology is destiny, that sexual difference is the essential difference between men and women, rather than the social constructs that have been built on the basis of that difference (Lury 1991: 95–108). Elizabeth Wilson sums up this dilemma succinctly: 'Not only is much fiction autobiographical; all auto-biography is in some sense fictional – the remembrance or the searching again for the "lost times" is never just an act of memory or research, but is inevitably a re-creation, something new' (Wilson 1988: 21).

With these reservations borne in mind, autobiography as a feminist methodological tool can serve to illuminate the processes of negotiation entailed in becoming a feminine subject. Contemporary feminist writings use autobiography to explore subject formation and generational change. For example, Liz Heron's edited collection *Truth, Dare or Promise: Girls Growing Up in the Fifties* (1985) presents a range of accounts from women who later became feminists; Carolyn Steedman's *Landscape for a Good Woman* (1986) explores theoretical constructions of working-class identity, emphasising their inability to address the complexities of her mother's life; and Valerie Walkerdine's *Schoolgirl Fictions* (1990) critiques and analyses her early working life as a primary school teacher. All explore the feminist axiom that the personal is political from a range of theoretical perspectives.

The aesthetic and philosophical problems raised by the feminist use of autobiographical writings pertain to a particular representational form of the self; this self clearly has some control over the forms (both aesthetic and institutional) through which such self re-presentation might occur. These writings illuminate aspects of what it means to experience life gendered female, but much of that experience continues to be unknown – not because, as Freud suggested, woman is a dark, unknowable other, but because women do not control the institutions and practices in which dominant discourses are developed. As Benner and Wrubel (1988) have pointed out, this is part of the problem faced by professional nursing; some of the expert knowledge of practising nurses is passed on orally because existing discourses are unable to convey certain kinds of information, partic-ularly that pertaining to intimate body care. Lawler (1991) locates the problem as an issue of power/knowledge, located quite specifically in an inability to discuss what nurses' work with patients actually involves because aspects of body care are privatised in 'civilised' society. This aspect of nurses' work, because there is no socially acceptable way to acknowledge it publicly, has been socially constructed on the basis of its invisibility, written off as 'women's work' and given low status in society (Lawler 1991: 219). Until recently, discussion or debate about nurses' body work has tended to be subsumed under the melodramatic rubric of 'tender loving care', with an implied devaluation of the skills involved in the art of caring. Within this overall context, the use of autobiographies and case studies of nurses' lives can be seen as part of a broader feminist and nursing endeavour to give voice and material substance to the experiences of women whose stories and knowledge remain untold and unknown in the public realm.

Framing others

The use of case studies is grounded in social science methodologies of empirical investigation and reportage; the technique has been of particular interest to feminists working in oral history, sociology and anthropology. As a feminist methodology, the case study approach has been exemplified by the work of anthropologists like Mascia-Lees, Sharpe and Cohen (1989) who stress the political applications of such studies in the fight for equal rights for minority groups and the formation of policy; it has also been used by oral historians such as Elizabeth Roberts (1986 and 1995) to insert knowledge of women's lives into the official fabric of the past.[34] In the context of this research, case studies are used to illuminate the relationship between images of nurses in general circulation and their impact on young women who became nurses during this period. Why did they decide to become nurses? What factors were responsible for their decisions? Case studies were seen as an appropriate means of investigation because it was important to try to obtain stories from those who were least likely to be represented in the existing histories of nursing. Issues of 'race', class and sexuality are absent from many conventional histories of nursing; the criteria for the selection of the case studies was that the person was likely to tell an untold story, one that official histories of nursing had not yet fully recorded.

In an illuminating article, Carolyn Steedman outlines an approach to the relationship between autobiography, biography and history which is a useful adjunct to the methodologies outlined briefly above. Steedman draws a parallel between the use of auto/biographical narrative in the construction of the self as a unitary subject of discourse, and the use of narrative in historical discourse to create a sense of linearity and progress. To quote her more fully:

> Written autobiography ends in the figure of the writer . . . the man or woman writing a book is the embodiment of something completed. History is a narrative that proceeds by the objectives of exhaustiveness and exception; and its central rhetorical device is this recognition of temporariness and impermanence. The fictionality of all these forms can be suggested . . . forms of writing that work by emplotment, by the use of figures and allusions, as well as by the presentation of their content, which is information about lives and times.

> (Steedman 1989: 110)

Autobiography, biography and history are used in this research to create a multi-layered narrative that ends not in the happy ever after of a stable nursing self but in a construction of nursing history that emphasises the gap between mediations of professional identity and lived experience.

2

THE POPULAR IMAGINATION

In this chapter the focus on fictional images follows my own growth pattern of the consumption of nursing images with one exception, that of film. The cinematic image of nursing was already in decline by the time I was old enough to go to the pictures, and I have few memories of nurses on the big screen. Sister Tutors in charge of recruitment during the late 1940s and 1950s, however, claim that the cinema was a major influence on the nurses they admitted to training.[1] Since it was this generation of nurses that in the 1970s was training me, I wanted to trace the images and ideologies of nursing that circulated during their formative years of training. Until the end of the 1940s, women formed the majority of cinema audiences in Britain (Thumim 1992). Nursing and hospital films of this period are therefore crucial to an understanding not only of the relationship between the cinematic image and the public perception of the nursing role, but the nursing profession's idealised view of itself.

The texts selected for detailed analysis are those that feature experiences of general nurses in training (rather than more general texts featuring nurses) and through those experiences, introduce readers and viewers to modern hospital life. Many of the stories feed an appetite for tales of female heroism, romance and mystery played out through life and death dramas against the backdrop of changes in health care. It was not only these romantic images of handsome young doctors and pretty, feminine nurses that fuelled a growing interest in stories about nursing and medicine; the texts fed a desire for knowledge, supplying contemporary medical facts and information. They offer maps of possibilities – the possibility of a certain kind of femininity, the possibility of a particular way of life, the possibility of professionalising (and earning money from) the 'womanly' skills associated with caring for people. They also hint at other possibilities – of gaining knowledge about the body and its functions, of healing, of life and death itself. In many of the narratives selected for study the stories map a journey from innocence to experience, the transition from girlhood to womanhood, through the process of nurse training. Nurses in these texts are central characters of narrative agency who both motivate action and around whom action happens. Central characters in fictional narratives are those that readers or viewers are most likely to align with, and therefore it is likely that when the central character is a nurse, alignment will lead to allegiance with that character and their situation.[2]

Reification and recruitment: images in post-war Britain

During and towards the end of the war the hospital system and the nursing profession were increasingly controlled by the state. An ethos of service and public duty pervaded notions of professional identity, perpetuating a vocational ideal of nursing as 'woman's mission'. Nursing was generally regarded as hard and dirty work, it was poorly paid and a sense of vocation was considered essential in order to be able to do it. British films and career novels for girls have a preoccupation with 'instruction', delivering education and information, an emphasis that is missing from many of the texts produced in later periods as popular images became increasingly influenced by North American models. There are a number of reasons why this was the case, some of which are dealt with below in relation to the films, the others in relation to career novels for girls. Only British films are considered in depth, although it is likely that cinema goers at the time would have been as familiar with Hollywood images of nurses and nursing as they were with the British product. Films like *The Citadel* (GB 1938) – made by MGM's British studio – and *Vigil in the Night* (US 1940) were written by the British writer A. J. Cronin but produced and distributed by American film companies. The movement of creative talent and personnel between the British film industry and Hollywood was common practice in the film industry at the time. Much has been written about the domination of British film distribution by American companies and the attempts by British companies, particularly J. Arthur Rank, to break into the American market.[3] The history of the British film industry throughout this period is not a particular concern here, but it is important to note that my division into British and American films is in some ways an arbitrary one from an audience point of view. In the late 1940s, there was considerable American investment in film production in Britain; the British film industry, as well as the British cinema audience, was heavily influenced by and familiar with the American product.[4]

In a similar way, it is difficult to draw clear lines of national specificity around two popular series of nursing career novels for girls in England, the *Sue Barton* and *Cherry Ames* books. Both were written by American writers but became widely available in Britain shortly after publication. Within a short space of time, they were available for loan on the shelves of local public libraries, and are still available today although now out of print; many women I have spoken to, from a wide variety of backgrounds and of different ages, recall reading these novels in their youth. Throughout the post-war period the popular image of nursing in Britain was heavily mediated by American fictions on the big screen and in books, but the lack of contextualising information in these texts created an image of nursing that seemed able to transcend barriers of national identity and other differences into an all-embracing ideal of white, middle-class femininity.

Nurses on screen

Some of the most thorough work on images of nurses in the movies has been undertaken by American scholars Beatrice and Philip Kalisch (1982b) who base their conclusions on content analysis of the nurse's role and function in over two hundred motion pictures produced between 1930 and 1979. Kalisch and Kalisch see the period between 1930 and 1945 as the heyday of positive images of nursing and nurses on the big screen. Throughout this period, nursing is portrayed as a worthy and important profession that enabled women to earn a living without compromising ideal feminine values, a depiction that developed alongside other new models for working women which were emerging in the depression years of 1930s America, a period of economic collapse and retrenchment. The only American feature length films that focused entirely on depicting contemporary nursing life were released during this time: *Night Nurse* (1931), *Once to Every Woman* (1934), *The White Parade* (1934), *Registered Nurse* (1934), *Wife, Doctor and Nurse* (1937), *Four Girls in White* (1939) and *Vigil in the Night* (1940). *The White Parade* (1934) is described as a realistic and sympathetic portrayal of the difficulties of becoming a nurse in a large hospital school. The story emphasises that not every woman is cut out to be a nurse, that nursing entails a life of hard work and little monetary reward but that it affords enormous personal satisfaction. At the end of the film, the heroine (*sic*) turns down marriage to a millionaire in order to continue working as a nurse. 'Marriage' to nursing is portrayed as equivalent to a religious vocation, a higher calling demanding both idealism and self-sacrifice. During the depression era the prevailing image of nursing on the screen changed from the self-seeking and consumerist values that had dominated the latter half of the 1920s, substituting ideas of self-sacrifice and virtue. Although all kinds of heroines were nurses, not one of them was a career nurse since careers were out of keeping with woman's legitimate destiny, marriage. By the mid-1930s, this view at least had undergone considerable transformation, with many of the later heroines determined to complete their nursing training (Kalisch and Kalisch 1982b: 607).

This analysis tells us very little about the relationship of American nurses and their professional institutions to the screen image of nursing, or why the sexualised image of some of the 1920s nurses becomes 'redeemed' during the depression. Kalisch and Kalisch's preference for the later films seems to be based on what they perceive as the 'realisticness' of the image and ignores the changing conventions of Hollywood cinematic practice, itself subject to rapid change which included both technological upheaval (the introduction of synchronised sound) and pressure to censor much of its output. What Kalisch and Kalisch mean when they point to the 'realisticness' of *The White Parade* is that this film upholds a particular set of meanings around the sign 'nurse' that are cognisant with their own nursing ideals and values. There is no ideological conflict between the filmmakers (in the broadest sense of the word) and the Kalischs' interpretation of the film, no gaps in shared understanding or knowledge.

The movement traced by the Kalischs between the 1920s, when nurses gave up their charitable work to marry wealthy spouses, and the mid- to late 1930s, when nurses abandon their matrimonial chances and 'sacrifice' themselves to nursing, neatly fits Richard Maltby's argument about the effects of censorship on narrative structure. He has convincingly argued that censorship, in the form of the Hollywood Production Code, was instituted in 1934 to protect dominant ideologies at a time when economic recession was straining popular belief in the American dream. His research shows that the Production Code Administration regarded narrative structure as a strategy for controlling meaning, and therefore particular narrative structures were used in the hope of reducing the possibility that contemporary audiences would develop oppositional identifications, beliefs and ideas (Maltby 1983). One of the adverse ideas that needed containing was the blatant display of consumerism through woman-centred spectacle as this was incompatible with the crisis of capital during the depression. Instead, there is a turn towards sacrifice films where women give up material wealth to be broke but happy. Kalisch and Kalisch do not comment on whether American nursing institutions capitalised on these 'positive' images to bolster recruitment during the depression years, leaving the relationship between these cinematic images and professional nursing's attitude to them open to speculation and further research.

Somewhat surprisingly, the largest group of films to feature nurses were detective and crime stories. The Mary Roberts Rinehart character Miss Pinkerton and Mignon Eberhart's Sarah Keate became popular screen nurse sleuths, working as private duty nurses for wealthy patients and becoming embroiled in the mysterious goings-on of the mansions' other occupants. These films usually ended with the nurse in the arms of a police detective boyfriend, but they were not primarily romantic stories and did not end in marriage, or for that matter with their leading characters going mad or dying – the fate of so many 1930s screen heroines. Kalisch and Kalisch like these films because the nurses display wit, mental acuity and courage; they are worldly wise, not easily taken in by outward appearances, and yet are portrayed as sympathetic and kindly women. There is little attention paid to actual nursing care in these stories – nursing work is depicted as administering medications, taking temperatures and delivering meals. By focusing on nurses as sleuths, a tactic used in the later *Cherry Ames* books, nurses are depicted as intelligent, rational women with logical powers of deduction who are capable of bravery, determination and forbearance. These films were very popular in the United States and were produced at the rate of one or two a year during the 1930s, but there is no researched evidence of their consumption and popularity in Britain.

With the entry of America into the Second World War, nurses on the screen assumed a patriotic, activist character which, according to the Kalischs, has never before or since been bettered (Kalisch and Kalisch 1982b: 608). Here, with the need for nurses at its most acute, Hollywood produced what film critic James Agee calls 'probably the most deadly accurate picture ever made of what war looks like through the lenses of a housewives' magazine romance' (Halliwell 1989: 934). Kalisch and Kalisch view this film, *So Proudly We Hail* (1943), as Hollywood's greatest tribute to the nursing profession. Apart from the film's being one of the top money makers of the year and academy award nominated, the Kalischs find the image overwhelmingly positive; several beautiful young nurses display self-sacrifice, heroism and stamina as they battle against overwhelming odds that culminate in the largest military surrender of troops in American history. The film emphasises their professional work and the *esprit de corps* that characterises their relationships with each other.

At the end of this period of their analysis Kalisch and Kalisch see the professional image of nursing emerging as a valuable one, with a set of requirements and standards for its practitioners. Nurse characters retained their romantic functions, but not to the exclusion of other activities: 'In this "golden age" of nursing films, women appeared able to practice nursing whilst pursuing personal lives. Even if marriage spelt the end of a nursing career, the career itself had mattered to these young women who recognised the value of their own contribution' (1982b: 609). This 'golden age' belongs to an era of cinema when women regularly formed more than 50 per cent of the audience for popular films, an era that Hollywood responded to and nurtured by producing films that would appeal to the female audience. Often referred to by critics and film scholars rather disparagingly as 'women's pictures', these films were crossed and informed by numerous genres, but always had as their defining characteristic a central character of narrative agency who was a woman. As feminist film critics have frequently pointed out, although these films depict a female view of the world the Hollywood production system is so thoroughly saturated with masculine values and ideals at all levels of the film-making process that 'women's pictures' are inevitably informed by male ideas and fantasies about women. Even when the director is a woman (in Hollywood this has always been a rarity), the generic constraints of mass film production and the need to compete with men in the system tend to militate against films which could be said to produce a viewpoint that is in any way radically different from the institutional (patriarchal) status quo. Nonetheless, as Haskell (1974) points out, the 1930s were marked by the comparatively large numbers of women screenwriters employed by the studios, and many of them scripted women's pictures.[5] It is therefore surprising to note that in the first group of films mentioned by Kalisch and Kalisch only one of them, *The White Parade*, is adapted from a female-authored novel and has a woman on the screenwriting team. Films about nurses in this era seem to be based on stories and scripts written by men, a situation reversed in Britain although there were fewer women working as scriptwriters.

Both the women's picture as a genre and the female audience began to decline from the 1930s on, for reasons that will be considered in more detail below. What it is important to note are two contextual factors that clearly affected the image of the nurse on the big screen at this time: the enforcement of the Production Code, effectively banning the development of 'the naughty nurse' image; and a cinema audience in which women were consistently in the majority and had to be catered for. These two factors, in the context of depression America, changed the image from one which either (re)presented the nurse as an icon of sacrificial womanhood or of sexual titillation and fantasy, to one where it was possible to practise nursing and enjoy a personal life as well.

Haskell (1974) points out that central to 1930s women's films is a notion of middle-classness that is not just an economic status, but a state of mind and behaviour. Women in these films, 'confronted by a range of options so limited that they might as well live in a cell', are dependent for their well-being and fulfilment on the social institutions of marriage and moth-erhood (Haskell 1974: 159–60). Arguably, by 'marrying' nursing, women who become nurses are equally dependent on these institutional constraints since the division of labour in health care echoes that of the normative ideal of the middle-class family with the doctor as patriarch, the nurse as mother and the patient as child (Gamarnikow 1978, Muff 1982b). Within American films about nursing in this period, the rigid moral code enforced on Hollywood by the Production Code tends to polarise female characters into 'good women' and 'bad girls'. Unlike in films of the 1920s, where it was possible for a 'bad girl' to redeem herself by becoming a nurse, in the 1930s nurses on the screen tend to polarise into 'good' and 'bad' types. Anne Karpf (1988a) points out these oppositional characteristics in *Vigil in the Night* (1940); 'badness' amounts to neglecting a patient to satisfy one's own needs (in this case leaving the bedside to make a cup of tea while caring for a sick child) with the result that the patient dies. Throughout the film, all the negative and critical comments about nursing are made by the Bad Nurse. Finally, she is punished for neglecting her duty; while nursing another child with smallpox, she contracts the disease and dies. The Good Nurse is rewarded with a doctor partner and is given the final lines of the film; 'We're here to serve, and if we do it well, we find pleasure, freedom, perfect freedom . . .' The moral of the film is clear: the wages of sin (in this case, putting one's own desires and needs before duty) is death; it is a woman's duty to serve others, both in the literal sense of performing services, and in the abstract sense of serving particular ideas, beliefs and values. Only through willing and obedient self-sacrifice and service can a woman hope to find happiness and fulfilment. Like Haskell's masochistic American housewife who is dependent on marriage for her identity, these women need the institutional context of nursing in order to function as 'good' characters.

In the 1920s, nurse characters had an iconic quality, embodying an essentially good, pure and untarnished femininity that set them apart from other female characters. This sign had the religious connotations of vocation and calling that were a part of nursing's mythic status. By the end of the 1930s, films were showing that it was possible for ordinary women to achieve that status but that it involved, as Kalisch and Kalisch point out, a great deal of self-sacrifice and determination. This is exactly the kind of sentiment that might be expected at a time when women were needed for nursing in ever greater numbers as the threat of war became reality, the Hollywood fiction factory serving patriarchal capitalism's hegemonic needs for women's low paid labour to service the war effort. Karpf notes that the release of *Vigil in the Night* in Britain came soon after an attempt to enhance the conditions, training and pay of nurses, and 'had the flavour of a recruitment drive' (Karpf 1988a: 209).[6] In British films about nursing, recruitment is a recurrent concern during war-time and its immediate aftermath.

British film products in the 1940s tended to fall into two categories labelled at the time by British producer Michael Balcon as 'realism and tinsel'. Robert Murphy uses Balcon's classification to examine the relationship between cinema and society, pointing out that the 1940s are considered by many film scholars to be the 'golden age' of British cinema not so much because of the numbers of films produced, but because of their realist aesthetics and their concentration on issues that particularly pertain to the British way of life (Murphy 1989). In British cinema history, this legacy of a uniquely 'British' style has traditionally been traced back to the documentary movement of the 1930s, and in particular to one man, John Grierson, who regarded cinema in much the same way that Lord Reith (head of the BBC) regarded British broadcasting; that is, its function was to inform, educate and entertain the masses, with the emphasis squarely placed on informing and educating. Film critics such as Dilys Powell and Roger Manvell and film producers like Michael Balcon welcomed the realist aesthetic as a progressive force that would 'wean people away from their dependence on unhealthy fantasies and help them to become more worthy and responsible citizens' (Murphy 1989: 1). There was the sense of a moral and political crusade attached to the realist film, a mission that had a class-based dislike and disapproval of what was then regarded as 'the vulgarity and crudity' of much popular culture, particularly in its imported American forms of movies and dance music. Other producers (but few critics) argued that what the public needed and wanted were escapist films that had nothing to do with the horrors and realities of war. Hence, the realism and tinsel metaphor – with films featuring nurses falling solidly into the 'realism' category, even though that 'realism' now feels distinctly stodgy, artificial and class-based.

The nursing profession was keen to boast of and maintain its middle-class credentials during this period, as it had in earlier decades. Throughout the 1930s, the professional wing of nursing under the auspices of the College of Nursing had tried to unite the different nursing factions, fighting a hard battle with the municipal hospital sector and its unionised workforce. Central to the College's philosophy was the idea of service, a 'no-strike' stance that was the cornerstone of their claim to professional rather than trade union status. The elite who ran nursing during this period, in the main the Matrons of the powerful London voluntary hospitals attached to university schools of medicine, were active in promoting their image of nursing to the public through articles in magazines aimed at middle-class readers, such as *The Lady* and *Zodiac*. It therefore comes as no surprise to find representatives of this select group acting in an advisory capacity to filmmakers wanting to depict nursing on the big screen. A combination of advice from those who sought every opportunity to reify their ideal of nursing as service and self-sacrifice with filmmakers using realist strategies produced a series of unexciting, didactic films that had the specific intention of boosting nursing morale and raising the levels of recruitment. Throughout the war-time period, documentary realism worked hand in hand with official propaganda to produce films such as *The Gentle Sex* (Auxiliary Territorial Service (ATS) training, GB 1943), *Millions Like Us* (munitions factory work, GB 1943) and *The Lamp Still Burns* (nursing, GB 1943) to encourage women to support the war effort. In the 1930s there had been strict moral and political censorship of films exercised by the British Board of Film Censors, controls that in war-time were changed and supplemented by the Ministry of Information who both advised on and proposed relevant filmic subjects. Films featuring nurses were amongst this latter group, made not for their entertainment value but to inform and educate the general public about nurse training in a vain attempt to alleviate the acute shortage of labour.

The writer Monica Dickens had considerable influence on the image of nursing at this time. Her popular autobiographical novel *One Pair of Feet* (1942), which tells of her early war-time experiences as a volunteer nurse, was used as the basis for a war-time recruitment film, *The Lamp Still Burns* (GB 1943).[7] The film's nursing adviser was the Matron of a major teaching hospital, the London, and, as with a number of feature films produced in war-time Britain, funding was provided by the government. The opening credits, presented against a background featuring a statue of Florence Nightingale with a suitably sombre classical musical score, announced the film's worthy intentions: 'A tribute to all those who nurse made with the assistance and collaboration of the Ministry of Health.'

What is surprising about *The Lamp Still Burns*, given the shortage of nursing labour at the time, is how little the class barriers have shifted or changed in the interests of reaching a popular audience. In *Millions Like Us* the aspirant working-class heroine (*sic*) Celia dreams of becoming a nurse while awaiting her call-up, but is drafted to work in an aircraft factory. Throughout the 1940s and the early 1950s, there are no depictions of working-class women as nurses on the big screen. In spite of the recruitment shortage and evidence that nursing's main pool of labour was drawn from shop girls and low grade clerks,[8] the nursing heroine of *The Lamp Still Burns* is a middle-class architect who gives up her profession and business partnership to train as a nurse. The underlying ideological message is that there are greater personal satisfactions to be gained from nursing than from entering male-dominated professions offering new opportunities for women. It is difficult, however, to envisage how the leading character, Hilary, might have offered a position of aspiration or allegiance for the majority of women in the cinema audience; nursing is portrayed as constant drudgery. Hilary spends more time in the sluice scrubbing dirty bedpans and equipment than caring for patients. As was usual in nursing films of this period, the patients are mostly men, many of them working-class; the problem of depicting a middle-class woman serving working-class women is avoided by omission. In this sense, the film projects a classical 'Nightingale' image of the profession, displacing issues of class and gender difference through the use of the 'angel' icon.

Stylistically, *The Lamp Still Burns* has many of the features of British realism that distinguished films of this period from their Hollywood counterparts. The film looks like a studio production, with each shot carefully measured and lit, but displays no expressive overtones in the lighting style or in the *mise-en-scène*.[9] Similarly, the acting is taut and underplayed, expressive close-ups are avoided and little use is made of musical underscore to enhance the emotional intensity of the action. This emphasises the spoken word as the supplier of the film's meaning, giving it a didactic quality; we are informed and instructed (and sometimes uplifted) by the dialogue, rather than emotionally swept along by the images and the music. Nonetheless, Rosamund John's character is convincing. Her determination to get what she wants, and to change the training system in the process, is an indication of changing attitudes about women's public role as nurses and their private role as wives. It is an admission that these spheres are not necessarily mutually exclusive for women, although both are framed within a bourgeois liberal humanist ideal of service.

Striking in its similarities to *The Lamp Still Burns* is a film produced in 1951 by the Crown Film Unit for the Ministry of Information, *Life in Her Hands*. Produced specifically with the aim of recruiting women to nursing, the film was distributed on all the major cinema circuits. Although a fictional film with a screenplay co-written by Monica Dickens, publicity billed it as a documentary; *Monthly Film Bulletin* describes the film as 'combining impersonal information with a personal fictional story' (1951 210, 18: 301). The central protagonist, Ann, has some similarities to Hilary in *The Lamp Still Burns*. Like Hilary, she is older than the usual age of entry to nurse training, arriving at her decision only after her husband's death in a car crash. As the driver of the car, she feels guilty and responsible for the accident; the 'fictional' content of the film is the story of Ann coming to terms with her feelings of guilt. Ann is from a very middle-class background, and is likewise warned by her family and friends of the long and difficult training she will have to undertake to become a nurse. Unlike Hilary, however, Ann is deemed to have a vocation by the Sister Tutor: she is a 'born' nurse, not someone who merely wants to do a useful and worthwhile job. The vocational element is much stronger in this film, in part signified by the nurses' uniforms with their flowing, veil-like caps. The overall impression continues to be one of 'closed orders', a community of women living a narrowly segregated life under a strict authoritarian regime.

The realist style of presentation earned this film its documentary label, but the scenes of hospital life are careful reconstructions of the actuality they represent. The 'fictional' sections of the narrative, which depict Ann's family life away from the hospital, are awkward, artificial and unconvincing. Considering the film was made with the sole intention of informing viewers about nursing work and has no romantic or other narrative interest, depiction of the work lacks detail. Only one sequence stands out, a montage that focuses on Ann's hands and facial expressions as she performs a number of routine nursing tasks. This tightly shot and edited sequence emphasises hand/eye co-ordination and concentration, creating an impression of skill and dexterity in the nursing process, but the patients on whom these tasks are performed are absent participants, background presences for the nursing drama performed on and around them. Again, no female patients are featured and the working-class male patients are infantilised, appearing as mischievous but otherwise harmless children. Other nursing characters veer towards caricature; one Sister is obsessed with weighing tea to check if the night nurses are using too much. Another, large chested and formal, warns her patients, 'You'll be dead before Christmas if you don't do what I tell you'. The dialogue in much of the film seems artificial, perhaps because too much emphasis is placed on presenting information at the expense of character development and plot.

In a personal telephone conversation with Miss H, former Sister Tutor in charge of nurse training at the Liverpool Royal Infirmary during this period, I asked her if she thought films like *Life in Her Hands* influenced nurse recruitment in any way. Her considered opinion was that these films did little to encourage girls into nursing; she thought that Hollywood-style films featuring famous nursing heroines such as Edith Cavell and Florence Nightingale were far more influential. By the mid-1950s, Anna Neagle had come to epitomise for professional nursing the vocational ideal and heroic commitment to the profession that many nurses sought to promote. In an article published in the *Nursing Mirror* shortly after her portrayal of the Matron in *No Time for Tears* (GB 1957) Neagle claimed that 'the portrayal of nurses has given me great personal happiness, and I am indeed gratified if the nursing profession has found my portrayals satisfying' (Neagle 1958). Neagle played Florence Nightingale in the only British biopic of her life, *Lady with the Lamp* (GB 1951), directed by her husband Herbert Wilcox. By this time, the actress and director duo were well established as makers of popular melodrama about the lives and loves of the aristocracy. Experts in patriotic nostalgia, in the 1930s they made films such as *Victoria the Great* and *Sixty Glorious Years* with Neagle playing Queen Victoria in the starring roles. By the 1940s, Neagle was one of the top British stars at the box office along with Margaret Lockwood, Phyllis Calvert, Celia Johnson and Ann Todd. By the time she came to play Nightingale, she had accrued a classy 'star persona': a set of audience expectations about her derived from previous performances, fan magazines, interviews and other public appearances (Thumim 1992). Neagle's persona was that of an upper-class English lady, a role that she played in her 'private' life as well as on the screen.

It is this persona that Neagle brings to the biopic of Nightingale's life in a worthy depiction that attempts to describe not only her experiences in the Crimea, but also her skills as an administrator and her romantic attachments and business connections to the men who assisted her in her aims and ambitions. The film has all the marks of an expensive quality production, with a lavish *mise-en-scène* set in the stately homes of England and large numbers of extras. Considerable pains were taken to construct a historically accurate biography, in part a response to the romanticised Hollywood biopic of Nightingale's life, *The White Angel* (1936), but the film still tends to lapse into sentimentality, particularly in the scenes where Nightingale is tending the injured soldiers at Scutari. Some emphasis is placed on Nightingale's dealings with the 'drunkards and prostitutes' who are the tenders of the sick until her programme of reform, substantiating a professional view of working-class women as irresponsible and vulgar and nursing as a career for well bred middle- and upper-class women.

Unlike Hollywood's image of Florence Nightingale in *The White Angel*, *Lady with the Lamp* attempts to present Nightingale's work throughout her long life, aspiring to project historical authenticity through extensive use of location shooting and excessive attention to period detail. In contrast, as the title suggests, *The White Angel* presents Nightingale as an iconic figure, tailored to suit prevailing notions of sacrifice in depictions of 1930s womanhood. Archetypal images of 'Woman' as bride, nurse and nun are merged in the *mise-en-scène* of the film through the use of costume, lighting and the placing of Nightingale (played by Kay Francis, an American actress with a 'classy' persona like that of Neagle) in the film frame. Her decision to nurse, for example, is presented as sudden and forceful, like a religious conversion. Nightingale (Francis) is dressed completely in white, with a dress and veil that are both bridal and religious in their connotations.[10] She announces her decision to nurse from a chair that looks like a throne, after a scene where she has expressed a yearning to be like Queen Victoria so that she could do a man's work and express a man's point of view (Hudson Jones 1988: 226). Visually placed as a queen on a throne, her face radiantly illuminated and wearing white robes, she presents an icon of white femininity that encapsulates sacrificial power and collapses the discourses of nursing and colonialism in a way that is similar to Nightingale's use of rhetoric (outlined in Chapter 1). Her representation as a 'white angel', a symbol of beauty and purity, reduces her whiteness to goodness at a level of universal abstraction that is removed from any racially specific context. This slippage, between 'whiteness' and 'goodness', and the explicit moral and aesthetic superiority implied in the image masks the socio-historical conditions on which such claims to superiority lie and the implicit power relations on which they were built.[11] In *Lady with the Lamp*, scenes that achieve a similar iconic effect through visualisation are, predictably, those where Nightingale walks amongst the sick with her lamp. Here, the effect is achieved through the signifying power of myth, a common code or shorthand that references popular knowledge of Nightingale's cultural status; the cluster of associations that the image conveys, such as self-sacrifice, humanity and endurance, have become naturalised as common sense and need no further explanation.[12]

In essence *Lady with the Lamp* conveys a worthy attitude to its subject that fails to re-kindle the spirit that inspired Nightingale's contemporary admirers and supporters. This is in part the result of a narrative that focuses on obtaining money, which in retrospect appears to be foregrounding a contemporary issue, the problems of funding the newly created NHS. In their attempt to portray a less idealised portrait of Nightingale's life, the filmmakers do little to disturb prevailing notions and ideological interpretations of her contribution to nursing history; the film is, perhaps, all the poorer because of this.

Finally, in conclusion to this cycle of films that instruct and educate about nursing, mention must be made of *White Corridors* (GB 1951), although it is primarily a film about a hospital and, unusually for the time, has a female doctor as its principal character. The film was adapted for the screen by two female screenwriters, Jan Read and Pat Jackson, from the novel *Yeoman's Hospital* by Helen Ashton. Stylistically, the film occupies an interesting space between the 'social problem' films of the 1940s, which attempted to portray the social conditions of working-class life, and the later 'Free Cinema' films, which extended the concept of a realist tradition in British cinema through their extensive use of location shooting.[13] *White Corridors* makes considerable use of location, setting the story against the backdrop of a provincial northern town which gives the film an aura of 'authenticity' missing in earlier films. Attention has been paid to depicting patients as characters from the town, placing the hospital within the broader context of the community it serves and cares for. The narrative trajectory of the film tells the story of an ambitious young doctor who wishes to work in a prestigious London hospital to further her medical career. This desire is complicated through her romantic attachment to a committed medical researcher, who wants to remain where he is. Although the doctors' professional and romantic lives form the backbone of the plot, with issues of female commitment to career and family values clearly foregrounded, the film has a number of other significant characters who play major roles, two of whom are nurses.

Education, information and entertainment are well balanced in this film, with the emphasis on contemporary issues in the NHS; unequivocal in its support of the value of the NHS, the film enacts several of the bureaucratic and procedural changes that have been introduced and debates how to prioritise the government's meagre budget allocation. Attention to the detail of contemporary debate extends to the portrayal of the nursing staff and their internal relationships with other hospital staff, an aspect of nursing life missing from both *The Lamp Still Burns* and *Life in Her Hands,* where the only other hospital workers are doctors. In this film, the class relationships between nurses, doctors and other workers form a clear hierarchy, with the nursing staff occupying a position somewhere in the middle. Although well-spoken, the nurses are less pretentiously middle-class than in other films; their comparatively inferior status is foregrounded in relation to the high status middle-class women who are either doctors themselves or engaged to doctors.

The nurses good-naturedly complain about the damage done to their hands by endless washing up in the sluice and the kitchen, and the damage done to their figures by an endless diet of suet pudding and stodge. Although the patients (both male and female) are treated as children by the nurses and class differences between them are apparent, patients are shown as characters who are sometimes co-operative and good-natured, but equally grumpy and difficult. The Sisters on the whole command respect because of their knowledge of disease patterns and treatments; Matron is a level-headed administrator who tries to improve the lot of her staff amidst competing claims on the hospital's tiny budget. Running a hospital is shown to require a complex set of skills and judgements shared between medical and nursing staff and their lay administrators.

Fraternisation between the medical and nursing staff is not permitted in working hours, and one nurse is sacked as a result of such a liaison. In a heated exchange with the Matron, she exclaims: 'You have no right to interfere in my private life . . . I suppose you want us all to grow into frustrated spinsters.' The Matron, a kindly woman, is visibly shaken and upset by this and has to make an effort to pull herself together. Nurses in this film are portrayed as human characters rather than embodiments of iconic ideals. Their work is shown to be hard but rewarding, and the Sisters in particular are shown to have repositories of knowledge that doctors draw on and use in their work. Different aspects of the various jobs in nursing are clearly depicted so that, unlike in other films of the time, an audience is informed not so much about nursing tasks (which are to some degree obvious) but about nursing skills – skills learnt through clinical observation and nursing practice.

In conclusion, this group of films presents professional nursing's reified ideal image in a style which claimed to present an authentic view of the world to the cinema audience. Somewhat surprisingly, it is the totally fictional *White Corridors* which now seems to represent the clearest image of nursing life, but at the time it was criticised for its shallow depiction of characters although it had 'a quality of professionalism rarely seen in British films' (*Monthly Film Bulletin* 210, 18: 294). The nursing image on offer in most of these films is one of youthful eagerness to take on a life of duty, counting it as a privilege to serve a great and noble profession. The young self-sacrificing 'angel' is juxtaposed with older, more experienced nurses who present imposing images of matriarchal authority. It is hard to avoid the conclusion that becoming a nurse in these films heralds the possibility of a personal transition from 'angel' to 'battleaxe', an anxiety that some of the nurses I interviewed remember experiencing. 'Battleaxes' were women to both fear and respect; many of them had dedicated their lives to nursing after losing their loved ones in the First World War, a conflict that wiped out a generation of young men. These women embody a vocational image of nursing often found in Victorian popular fiction, women who had turned to nursing as a means of displacing thwarted sexual desire (Maggs 1983). During the Second World War and its immediate aftermath, this image had some resonance; Ann, for example, in *Life in Her Hands* is narratively placed as a widow searching for a substitution for her loss.

Janet Thumim points out that nursing figures as one of the few significant occupations amongst female characters in films of this period, only outstripped by the numbers of maids and performers of various kinds. Even so, nurses feature in only four popular films of the mid-1940s, ten in the mid-1950s with this number down to zero by the mid-1960s. In a comparative analysis of women's occupations featured in women's magazines, Thumim notes that the medical and caring professions are mentioned more than any other category, with nursing featuring as the most important group. Thumim concludes that the routine presentation of women on the screen throughout this period severely limited the career prospects of female audience members, who were 'more likely to find their horizons broadened in contemporary women's magazines than they were among the images of their celluloid sisters on the screen' (1992: 111–12). It has to be concluded then that there is little evidence that feature films significantly contributed to public perceptions of nurses and nursing throughout this period, in spite of the profession's and the government's belief that this was the case, and their attempts to use film as a vehicle for recruitment.

The use of feature films was complemented by the development of a range of 16 mm films that could be hired to show in schools, but whether any of these efforts increased recruitment levels seems unlikely. In a study that examined the effects of a recruitment film on the attitudes of school leavers towards nursing as a career, Jeffery (1950) concluded that there were no significant changes in attitudes as a result of the film, either in the immediate aftermath of watching the film, or six months later. Generally there was a dislike of the sight of blood, sick people and suffering, leaving home, night duty, studying, discipline and hospital work. Those who wanted to nurse were mainly interested in nursing children and had some direct experience of hospitals through their relatives. This general antipathy amongst Britain's school leavers led to a marked increase in attempts to recruit nurses from overseas.

Career books for girls

From the 1940s onwards, nursing career books for girls grew rapidly in popularity reaching a highpoint in the late 1950s and early 1960s.[14] A number of series were in circulation by the early 1960s, many of which were available from public libraries;[15] the most popular of these seem to have been the *Sue Barton* books written by Nurse Helen Dore Boylston.[16] *Sue Barton: Student Nurse* was first published in North America in serial format in *The Atlantic Monthly* in 1937: it appeared in book format in Britain in 1939;[17] six sequels followed at regular intervals. The books remain in circulation, although at the time of writing this book they are out of print.[18] Oxford University Press brought out the *Bunty Brown* books in the early 1940s as part of their career series aimed at young people aged 11 and upwards; the three books cover the three years of student nurse training. *Bunty of the Flying Squad* is the third book in the series, first printed in 1943.[19] The story creates a vivid impression of the changing class structure of British society during the war years. The hospital is based in a small town in southern England with a rural hinterland. Bunty presents an ideal image of professional nursing's favoured candidate for training; she is introduced on the back cover flap as 'a friendly, human little soul ... a constant source of warmest sympathy and practical help'. The daughter of a rural clergyman, she has experienced a childhood devoid of material riches but rich in cultural capital. She therefore has no difficulty communicating with the rich (the medical squirearchy in the form of Sir Ramsey and wealthy local business-men) or the poor (rural peasants and working-class 'rogues' with hearts of gold). Bunty endears herself to the rich by recognising their humanity and loneliness; money only brings happiness if it is socially useful. The pater-nalistic values of the traditional aristocracy are favourably contrasted with the poor taste and selfish behaviour of Mr Button, a self-made man who represents the 'new money' of the changing social order:

> 'Begging, eh?' he said. 'I never give money indiscriminately.'
>
> Marietta's eyes met Felton's [the butler]. How different in the old days, when Mr. Trevithen found it hard to refuse the most drunken tramp. Mr. Button frowned.
>
> 'That will do, Felton,' he snarled. 'I will show these two young women out'.
>
> (1959: 24)

Apart from the nurses, most of the women are the wives of peasants or unmarried spinsters; many of them are servants. The only wealthy woman in the text is depicted as a spoilt child, her attitude to poorer women one of condescension. Working-class women are depicted as coarse and vulgar but, like their menfolk, have hearts of gold:

> Mrs Gilbert had been accustomed to praise and admiration all her life – for her beauty and her delicate air in her youth, for her posi-tion and her money in her older years. But she had never been prouder of any compliment than when Mrs Hobbs, so reminiscent of her old Nannie, only a much more vulgar edition, called her a 'blinking old sport'.
>
> (p. 163)

Nursing skills are presented as ideal preparation for marriage, the training naturalised as suitable preparation for adult life as a wife and mother; by the end of the book, Bunty and her best friend are ready to marry at the same time as passing their final examinations and qualifying as nurses. Amongst the jobs that nurses do – sorting and folding linen, scrubbing equipment – preparing food and administering treatments are treated as prime skills. This world pre-dates antibiotics; patient recovery is shown to depend as much on good nursing care as on medical skills:

> 'I must congratulate you, Nurse. She's done well, hasn't she, Sister?'
>
> Roberta flushed with pleasure. Sister's kind eyes were on her too.

'She nearly made herself ill with worry at first, Sir Ramsey,' she said. 'But once over that, she's nursed her patient very well and done me credit, I think.'

Sir Ramsey, who thought the credit belonged to him, frowned at that, but a stumble from Harry diverted him.

(p. 57)

All the nurses, including the Matron and Sisters, are depicted as kindly, intelligent women; in contrast, the males (and doctors in particular) are sulky children who have to be pampered and humoured, their egos constantly supported by female deference:

Sir Ramsey took no notice. He was in a perverse mood and inclined to be jealous . . .

'These figures aren't correct', he said at last, in triumph. Roberta and Christine, who had so anxiously checked them, looked at him in dismay.

'You're fourpence out', he jeered.

Roberta was certain that they were not, but upon Matron's hinting to her to desist she did not argue the point, and thus gained a valuable lesson in the management of men.

(p. 29)

In contrast Bunty Brown and her nursing companions are able to transcend class differences; their range of backgrounds – one is Lady Marietta Power, the daughter of a Duke – present a small community of women united in a common cause to help the war effort by fighting to maintain standards of nursing care on the home front. Class and gender relations are foregrounded in British nursing stories for girls; based on mild adventure formats, the books negotiate a deferential, white middle-class femininity in which nursing is a 'natural' extension of womanly caring skills. Far less didactic than the films, the books present nursing as a job where learning about oneself through interaction with others equips those who train as nurses to deal with a wide variety of people and situations.

The Sue Barton and Cherry Ames characters are enduring cultural artifacts; created for a popular juvenile audience in the 1940s and 1950s, they seem to have achieved the kind of popularity that is in some ways equivalent to that of well-known characters of detective fiction. Re-reading the *Sue Barton* books after a period of some twenty-five years, I am struck by two immediate reactions before reading more than a couple of pages. The first is how familiar the stories seem to be (even though I do not think I read all the books, I was a committed *Cherry Ames* fan); the second is their similarity to doctor/nurse romances. I preferred the *Cherry Ames* books because they are primarily mystery stories with investigative thriller

48

narratives. What I did not remember about either series (if I ever knew) was that they were written by North American authors, and are about North American nurses and nursing. The female 'heroines' of these novels have that peculiar mix of characteristics which I now see as redolent of so much American writing for girls of that time – a combination of an adventuring, pioneering spirit with a determination to get what you want, yet with a preparedness to serve others and find it a pleasurable, enjoyable task. The writer of the *Sue Barton* series, Helen Dore Boylston, was a nurse for many years. She began her training at the age of 18 at the Massachusetts General Hospital in Boston in 1913; by the end of the First World War, she was a member of the Harvard medical unit for duty overseas with the British Expeditionary Forces. She later joined the American Red Cross, serving for two years in Poland and the Balkans before returning home to the Massachusetts General Hospital, where she taught nose and throat anaesthesia. A writer friend read her war diary and sent it to the *Atlantic Monthly*, where it was published in serial form; this was the beginning of a new career as a professional writer.

In spite of my personal preference for the *Cherry Ames* books, these are now less visible than the *Sue Barton* series and have not been reprinted in Britain since the 1960s, when they were brought out in hardback. There is less information available about the writers, Helen Wells and Julie Tatham, who between them produced at least sixteen books between the early 1940s and the late 1950s. Even so, these books were undoubtedly popular – *Cherry Ames Flight Nurse* was reprinted in Britain five times between 1956 and 1963; as a contribution to this project, several friends donated me copies which were given to them in the early 1960s.[20]

What interests me in these texts is their ideological function in relation to girls who were on the threshold of 'becoming women'; I remember that at the time I was reading these books 'becoming a woman' was at the forefront of my mind. My mother's only guidance in this matter was to give me a small pamphlet with a picture of a young woman holding a baby on the front. It was called, appropriately enough, *You're Becoming a Woman*, and described with the aid of diagrams the physical processes and changes in bodily appearance that would transform me from adolescence to maturity. But what sort of woman was I to become? In the period before my life became dominated by other adolescent interests, I read a great many mystery and romance books. For me, these books were landscapes of possibilities, maps to guide me through an unknown terrain. This aspect of pre-teenage reading is analysed by feminist researchers such as Linda Christian-Smith (1988) and Penny Tinkler (1995), who claim that cultural products present young readers with imaginative resolutions to the relations between the sexes and are productive of certain subject positions for them.[21] Their studies do not encompass career novels like the *Sue Barton* books, ostensibly about work, about the material world, which nonetheless use similar tropes and narrative formats to teenage romance texts. This combination of career and romance tends to sustain, at the imaginary level, the division of labour in health care, reinforcing what Gamarnikow (1978) has identified as the patriarchal familial structures inscribed in the relationship between medicine and nursing. Becoming a nurse in these books is about taking on a particular feminine identity, one that aligns nursing skills with wifely skills. Like other medical romances, such as those produced by Mills & Boon, the *Sue Barton* books in particular link working life and personal life through relationships with medical men. Because the heroines of these books invariably marry doctors, the difference between work in the public sphere as a nurse and work in the private sphere as a wife is subsumed through the discourse of heterosexual relationships. The hospital becomes a macrocosm of home life; doctors are fathers and husbands, nurses wives and mothers, and the patients their children.[22]

A clear example of this is found in *Sue Barton: Staff Nurse*, the sixth book in the series. Sue, married to the head of a small country hospital and bored at home with her three small children, feels that she is wasting her valuable skills and decides to return to work. This causes some consternation amongst the staff on the ward she is allocated to, for not only is she the boss's wife but she was also formerly nurse-in-charge of the hospital and had established the training school for nurses. Sue's best friend Kit, who trained with her and is her inseparable companion, is superintendent of nurses. Between them, Sue and Kit are 'ideal types' of nurse, each of them representing the particular aptitudes and skills that different areas of nursing work demand. Whereas Sue is presented as a practical nurse who excels in her contact with patients, Kit is a skilled manager who is responsible for the training and discipline of junior nursing staff. However, junior medical staff are totally outside her jurisdiction. One consequence of this division of duties and responsibilities is that a junior nurse has to be punished for a doctor's misdemeanour even though she is powerless in the situation, and Kit knows this is unfair. The incident centres on a romantic entanglement between a student nurse and her doctor boyfriend; messing about in the hospital dining room, he picks her up and carries her off. Although the powerlessness of the student is obvious (we already know Frank to be considerably bigger and taller than her), nursing management feel obliged to punish the nurse with suspension because she has set a bad example to other students. Not to do so might lead to a breakdown of hospital discipline amongst 'irresponsible students', who might see this as a green light for further misdemeanours with the medical staff. Placed in the position of having to treat a student unfairly, our resourceful 'girls' Kit and Sue decide to solve the problem by playing a trick on the doctor. His 'violently masterful' response to their challenge and subsequent proposal of marriage to the student is exactly the response Kit and Sue want and expect. An institutional problem, the disciplining of doctors to respect their nursing colleagues as equals in the public sphere of work, is resolved by emotional manipulation. Kit knows that she cannot 'punish' the doctor, she has no power to do so, and to complain to the medical hierarchy about a display of 'boyish high spirits' would only demean her. She uses subterfuge (her feminine wiles!) to get what she wants, rather than any kind of public, institutional action that would disturb the existing power relations. Nursing's subordination to medical power is naturalised in the narrative, accepted and circumvented, leaving the structural relationships between nurses and doctors intact.

In these books, the public and potentially political sphere of hospital work is articulated as the shared personal space of a small tightly knit group of female friends. Initiation into the nursing profession is an initiation into a small group or cohort which occupies a particular position within a rigid professional hierarchy. A major aspect of this initiation is the donning of the nurses' uniform, a process that exposes a private world of unwritten professional codes and rules, many of which are expressed in the complex signification of the uniform itself. An analogy is suggested between the public presentation of the private self in the everyday world through wearing certain kinds of clothes and the presentation of the public self in the world of work through wearing the nursing uniform. In the public presentations of the private self, we are given detailed descriptions of the clothes and make-up that Sue and her friends select for every social occasion, whether a walk in the country or a night at the theatre. As well as demonstrating how to dress as a young respectable middle-class single woman, the reader learns about lifestyle and attitudes. In the public sphere of work, a woman's attitude to her role as a professional nurse is judged by her personal appearance; nurses who wear their uniform incorrectly or their hair in the wrong style are described as 'untidy' and 'too casual' and defined as problems. The way these young women look, both on and off duty, is taken axiomatically to signify their attitude to their work and to the profession.

This preoccupation with appearances extends to fetishistic descriptions of the nurses' uniform: 'tiny crinoline cap with a black velvet band around a frilled base perched at a slight angle on smooth brown hair. White uniform, white shoes, white stockings and Eton collar were immaculate' (Dore Boylston, *Superintendent Nurse*: 9). The uniform is also a fashion item, the way the hat is worn at a particular angle negotiating the boundaries between the private self, nursing identity and the wider discourse of femininity and fashion manifested in contemporary ideas about clothes and how to wear them. As Dorothy Smith (1988b) cogently points out, fashion images are articulated around other meanings of the feminine such as particular virtues and resistances; femininity is a historically specific phenomenon whose articulations change over time. The nurses' uniform bears the traces of these changing virtues and resistances, inscribing on the bodies of those who wear it the ghosts of nursing foremothers and the relationship of those ghosts to contemporary professional ideals and values.

In the *Sue Barton* books, this foremother is indisputably Nightingale, a British nursing heroine, in spite of the American origins of the author.[23] Direct references to Nightingale and veiled hints refer to a past that is never articulated in historical terms, creating an aura of mythic deification around the Nightingale image. In *Student Nurse*, the first book in the series, Nightingale's presence is fully evoked through the memories of a very elderly patient who served as a drummer boy in the Crimean war. His memories of Nightingale as a 'lovely slim and gentle young thing' are a clear distortion of the known facts of history, but work at an emotive level in the text, emphasising self-sacrifice even to the point of death. For young women reading these books, the potency of this martyred image is reiterated by an incident immediately following this encounter, where Sue almost dies trying to save a patient's life.[24] It is this emphasis on Nightingale and Nightingale values in nursing which enabled the books to become cross-cultural artifacts.

Descriptions of clothes in these texts, and of uniforms in particular, are heavily value-laden. These values are re-articulated through the transforming process of putting on the uniform, and with it, a traditional ideal of professional identity. The student nurses in these stories are measured against this ideal, their success or failure as nurses depending on their ability to become more (or less) like the model nurses Sue and Kit, who are set up as complementary opposites both in terms of their appearance 'types' (red head, brunette) and as working 'types' (practical skills, management skills). In addition, as readers we are constantly presented with little descriptive homilies that remind us of the personal qualities needed to be 'good' women and successful nurses: '. . . she had that gift, supposedly common to all good writers or actors, of projecting herself into the interests and feelings of another person. It is a gift also common to good nurses, good friends – and good wives' (*Superintendent Nurse*: 54). The textually mediated discourse of femininity naturalises empathy as a female attribute and quality.

The books function much as sentimental novels functioned in the nineteenth century, presenting moral messages of self-abnegation to a readership on the threshold of womanhood, subjecting the reader to ideals of nursing and femininity which in the 1950s recruitment literature are encapsulated in the word 'service'. But for Sue Barton and Kit nursing is not only a matter of serving but a way of living. The books present nursing as an on-going, developing career that mirrors the development of Sue's romance, her marriage and the birth and growth of her children. There is no distinction between work and personal life, only an all-encompassing narrative that weaves a seamless web of interlaced experiences. This lack of separation naturalises the relationship between nursing and femininity, creating an image of female identity that is unproblematic and static, a

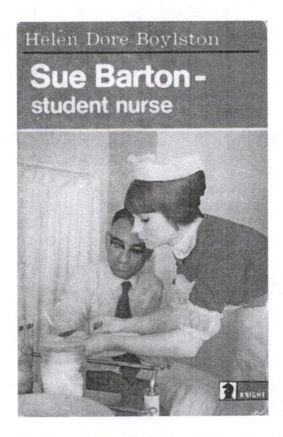

Figure 2.1(a) Cover, *Sue Barton: Student Nurse*, Helen Dore Boylston (Knight Books, 1971)

white heterosexual middle-class ideal against which women are judged as deviant or 'other' if they are different. 'Race' is an invisible absence; whiteness is naturalised as unexceptional, the normal state of affairs, difference a peculiar attribute of working-class patients from the slums.[25] Patients are treated much in the way that Sue treats her children, emphasising their infantile dependence and the 'innate' womanliness of nursing work. As career novels for girls, the books subject readers to an image of work against which they can measure themselves not in terms of intellect or ability, but in terms of how they look, what class they come from, and how they measure up to nursing's feminine ideal. These stories present a reactionary, old-fashioned view of what it means to be a working woman. Within the melding of the public and private discourse at this particular point in history there is, however, some space for recuperation. In the 1940s and 1950s, giving up work on marriage was virtually mandatory for

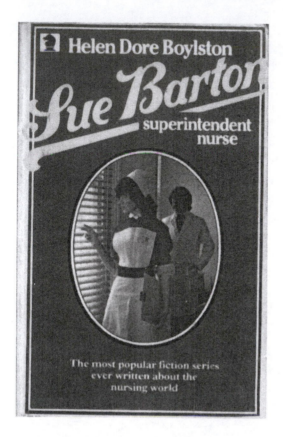

Figure 2.1(b) Cover, *Sue Barton: Superintendent Nurse*, Helen Dore Boylston (Knight Books, 1981)

most middle-class women, but Sue Barton manages to combine marriage with a career, and through this juggling act perhaps symbolises the possibilities for those (young middle-class white women) becoming nurses in the future.

In a different way, the *Cherry Ames* stories also provide a model of nursing as a career that was perhaps more dynamic at the time than appears to be the case now. The image of nursing presented initially appears more attractive; there is less emphasis on notions of respectability and appearance, hierarchy and discipline, the accent falling on the range of possibilities inherent in the nursing situation itself. The titles of the books, rather than mapping out a career path in different fields of nursing work, present some eighteen venues for nursing, from hospitals to ships, mountains and the army. Structured as mysteries where Cherry Ames always plays a leading role in solving the problem, the books seem to have more in common with the nurse detective movie series of the 1930s than with the *Sue Barton* books.

Articulations of the relationship between nursing and femininity are also rather different. Cherry Ames wears both powder and nail varnish on duty – in the Barton books an indication of working-class vulgarity, but here a sign of glamour and sophistication. There is less detail about clothes and uniform, and much more about the actual work that Cherry is doing; the job of nursing itself sounds interesting, rather than the lifestyle of being a nurse. In *Flight Nurse*, for example, we are told that Cherry has learnt to arrest haemorrhages, dress wounds, adjust splints, administer plasma and give shock treatment whilst flying at different altitudes without a doctor present. There seems to be more reason in these texts for discipline and self-sacrifice, and descriptions of the work, although at times lapsing into sentimentality, do demonstrate a range of skills accompanied by both a caring nature and strength of mind. The investigative format presents Cherry Ames as intelligent and able to act on her own initiative. Cherry was certainly the epitome of my young woman's dreams of the feminine ideal – beautiful, intelligent and adventurous, living a life where she was foot-loose and fancy free, much sought after by young men, but not in need of a permanent partner, even in the closing pages of the book.

In other ways though, the image of femininity Cherry represents is still that of the good girl, someone who wants to please because pleasing others is the key to popularity, and therefore to personal happiness. Although she is resourceful and uses her own initiative, Cherry also unquestioningly obeys doctors' orders, and treats patients like naughty children when they break hospital rules. Nursing as a profession seems far less powerful than in the Barton books, perhaps because its contextual relations are described more fully. In *Cherry Ames: Night Supervisor*, although Cherry is in charge of the nursing staff, it is clear that she is employed by a chief medical officer who runs the hospital and has the power to hire and fire nursing staff. Nursing is depicted as a job rather than a profession, a worthwhile and satisfying job, but one in which the notion of service is limited to serving the needs of male doctors and male patients. The opportunities afforded by nursing training are those of travel and adventure rather than a life of dedication to professional ideals and values, but the metaphors of travel and adventure obscure the underlying ideological implications in the text of nursing's associations with colonial and military objectives.[26]

Throughout the post-war period and into the early 1950s, the fictional images of nursing available to the general public in films and books tended to emphasise a white, middle-class feminine ideal of nursing. In their different ways, these fictions re-articulate notions of sacrifice common in women's films of the 1930s and 1940s, accommodating new ideas about

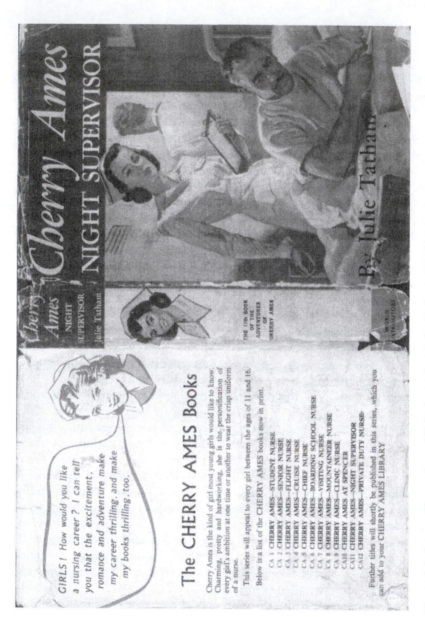

Figure 2.2 Cover, *Cherry Ames: Night Supervisor*, Julie Tatham (World Distributors, 1961)

the relationship between marriage and career prevalent in post-war culture. While some fictions, like the *Cherry Ames* series, use nursing as a background for adventure stories and mysteries, many of them reify the idealised, 'angel' image during a period of rapid upheaval and change. Attitudes to nurses and nursing amongst the public at large became much more ambivalent from the mid-1950s; cultural products mediate a sense of dissatisfaction and generalised unrest (what cultural analyst Raymond Williams refers to as a 'structure of feeling'[27]) that materialised with the election of the Labour government in the early 1960s.

Irreverence and romance: the 1950s and 1960s

The reification of Nightingale values encapsulated in the nursing films of the early 1950s was followed by a rapid shift in style towards films which treated nursing characters as melodramatic heroines or as objects of parody and derision. The late 1950s and early 1960s saw a proliferation of British films about hospital life on the big screen. In particular, the popular and successful '*Doctor*' films followed the life and loves of a newly qualified medic in a lighthearted look at the British medical establishment, and the '*Carry On*' series found in hospital life an ideal location for lampooning the British establishment and its paternalistic values. Within the 'Carry On' format in particular, nurses became an easy target for 'toilet' humour as well as a generative source of it. For the first time, working-class nurses were depicted on the screen, represented as busty sex objects (Barbara Windsor in *Carry On Doctor* GB 1968) or as authoritarian targets of derision (Hattie Jacques in *Carry On Matron* GB 1972), but they were not passive. Joan Sims' depiction of a down to earth (working-class) nurse commenting, 'What's all this fuss about such a little thing then', as she peers under the bedclothes on the pretext of preparing a male patient for theatre, exemplifies the irreverent approach of these films. Nurses are no longer nice middle-class girls coolly detached from the bodily functions of their patients, but working-class women who talk in saucy sexual innuendoes to their physically helpless male charges. They are not the asexualised, virginal 'nice' girls of earlier films, but pneumatic busty blondes who delight in causing 'out of control' physical responses in incumbent male patients. The image of professional nursing authority encapsulated in the 'battleaxe' is perhaps the cruellest of these stereotypes, with Hattie Jacques frequently playing the frustrated Matron or the Sister who is too old, too plain and too fat for sex. While younger nurses demonstrate hearty sexual appetites and cheeky intelligence, for older females, no longer sex objects, sexual desire is depicted as laughable and grotesque. Ineffective in their ability to attract men, senior nurses are often depicted as institutional puppets, petty tyrants without authority who play out their frustrations on powerless junior nurses and patients.

These filmic images stand in stark opposition to earlier ones, and can certainly be seen as derogatory of professional nursing values, but situated in a film genre that aims to poke fun at middle-class prudery and restraint, they follow in a tradition of music hall humour where the working man mocks those who seek to order and control his life. Created to entertain the young male audience who formed the bedrock of cinema's clientele by the late 1950s,[28] they mock not only the prudery of middle-class female sexuality, but the impotency of middle-class medical men. Their critique is class-based, aimed at mocking both middle-class propriety and working-class mores. Within the ensemble playing of the regular cast, Kenneth Williams invariably plays the part of the chief medical officer as a middle-class sexual impotent, while working-class patients (particularly those played by Sid James) are always depicted as worldly wise and sexually voracious.

The hospital was a popular venue for *Carry On* films, no doubt because of its suitability as a setting for generating comedy based around bodily functions and sexuality. Much of the humour lies in the way in which the institution is unable to control the actions and reactions of physical bodies through its timetables, regimes and regimentations. As Marion Jordan points out, the characters and the humour are those of the most demotic types of fiction – the comic postcard and the bar-room joke. The jokes are not only obscene, but they express a very masculine view of the world, where the castrating mother-in-law is always the wife's mother, sexual desirability (however much parodied) is most commonly female, sexual desire and potency most commonly male (Jordan 1983: 318).

The status of these films as popular (working-class) entertainment has been reflected in the lack of serious consideration given to them in histories of the British cinema, even though they were the top box office films of their day. It is only in recent years that they are acknowledged as part of a cultural heritage that lampoons traditional class values, hierarchical structures and British 'restraint'.[29] The films can be read as an early indication of the consumer critique of medical services which becomes much more pronounced in the 1970s, the first sign of public unease with medical power that questions the basis of bio-medical authority, the powerlessness of patients and their automatic regression to infantile status. The male working-class patients wreak havoc in the institution by refusing to obey orders, pointing out in the process how the sterile environment creates impotency amongst medical men and petty authoritarianism and sexual frustration amongst the nursing staff. In later films in the series such as *Carry On Doctor* (GB 1968), female patients do appear but the action is still centred on the antics of male patients, avoiding by omission the problem of how to generate humour for the predominantly male audience from female to female nurse–patient encounters.

Amidst the lighthearted capers of the *Doctor* films, and the lampooning *Carry Ons*, there were a few films that took nursing explicitly as their subject matter. Three in particular stand out as significant explorations of nursing life: *The Feminine Touch* (1956) follows the training of five nurses at a major London teaching hospital, *No Time for Tears* (1957) explores the nursing of sick children, and *Twice Round the Daffodils* (1962) follows the progress of a group of patients in a long-stay TB sanatorium. The most noticeable change in *The Feminine Touch* and *No Time for Tears* from their 1950s 'drama documentary' predecessors is a tendency towards melodrama and sentimentality that is heightened by colour cinematography and high production values in the presentation of the filmed image. The uniform, with its belted waist and billowing apron, was ideally suited for subtle adaptation towards the 'New Look' that became fashionable during the1950s; the result is a nursing workforce at the peak of its glamour on the British screen.

Attributed to designs by Christian Dior, the 'New Look' heralded a return of constricting fashion after the more relaxed styles of war-time, creating clothes that were difficult to move about in. Cone-shaped breasts, corseted abdomens and waspish waists exaggerated a female body form draped in long full skirts accompanied by pointed-toe shoes with slim heels. Read by some cultural critics as a sign of post-war nostalgia for Edwardian feminine values, 'New Look' fashion eschewed the 'masculine' tailored suits and smart dresses that had led fashion throughout the 1940s in favour of an abundance of soft flowing fabrics and dainty accessories.[30] *The Feminine Touch* exemplifies how the 'New Look' is part of a wider discourse on femininity that re-situates women in the domestic sphere, even though women (and in particular, married women) were recruited into the general workforce in increasing numbers from this period (Wilson 1980). Although the film is ostensibly about becoming a working woman, the articulations between fashion and femininity signify a contradictory attitude that places female nurses securely at the altar beside their male medical colleagues rather than at the bedside of their patients.

Following in the pattern set by *The Gentle Sex* (GB 1943) which portrayed seven different 'types' of young women undergoing their war-time ATS training, *The Feminine Touch* tells the story of five young women becoming nurses and learning to accept each other's differences in the process. These differences are articulated around notions of gender, class and nationality with 'Irishness', 'working-classness' and 'upper-classness' used to offset the 'norm' of white bourgeois 'Englishness' encapsulated in the two leading characters. The five stereotypes can be summarised as the beautiful, naive blonde (Susan), the sophisticated, worldly wise brunette (Pat), the plain ex-public school girl (Ann), the fiery red-haired Irish beauty (Maureen) and the untidy working-class girl from the East End of London (Liz). Needless to say, following the fashionable trend for blonde, busty female stars in the 1950s, the story focuses on the glamorous blonde Susan (a Sue Barton for adults) with the brunette Pat (Kit the administrator) in

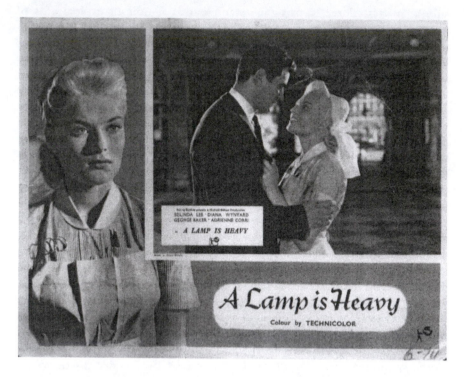

Figure 2.3 Publicity poster for *The Feminine Touch* (dir. Pat Jackson, 1956; adapted from the American novel *A Lamp is Heavy* by Sheila Mackay Russell and released in the USA with that title)

a strong supporting role. Susan manages to exemplify the 'New Look' both in her uniform when on duty and in mufti when off, whereas Pat presents a more traditional '1940s' image of the career girl in her smart fitted suits. Although they are opposite 'types', this does not stretch beyond superficial appearances; both women marry doctors, so obviating the need for any serious consideration of their nursing abilities or their career prospects. Pat, although she looks like a career girl, is scathing about nursing as a vocation; she has left a job in the city to take up training because she wants to find a doctor husband and marries an older man while still in training. Through this narrative device the film questions the restrictive rules and regulations surrounding the marriage of nurses even though Pat, for reasons of verisimilitude, gives up her own career to care for her husband.

Where this film forms an interesting comparison with the earlier 'recruitment' and information films is in its actual depiction of nursing work. Here, and in *No Time for Tears* which followed it a year later, nurses are seen less on the wards attending to their patients or in sluices scrubbing the bedpans, and more in the ward kitchens where they engage in preparing food, often for doctors. Narratively it is indicated that they are feeding the doctors at some considerable risk to themselves, since the food they are using has been provided for the patients and they are stealing it. Consorting with the doctors and squabbling with other nurses over who should be privileged enough to feed them is a major activity in these films, rather than interaction with the patients or the demonstration of nursing skills. In *The Feminine Touch*, a similar montage sequence to the one used in *Life in Her Hands* (1951) shows the busy-ness of nursing work depicted through a series of faces in close-up calling for a nurse, with patients intercut between Sisters. All the voices and faces are female. But in the narrative structure of the film it is the doctors who command nurse attention; senior nurses and patients are obstacles that have to be overcome to meet their needs. Doctors are depicted doing many of the minor tasks for the patient that, in earlier films, were the province of nurses; her role is diminished, confined to the kitchen and caring for doctors. Nursing is shown as a suitable training for a woman's 'real' work in life, looking after her (doctor) husband and children. The films depict a fantasy of femininity based on 'New Look' fashion and kitchen-centred caring. Even the voices contribute to this domestic ideal, with shrill tones of little girl eagerness and close-ups of trembling lipped femininity contributing to the overall impression of soft focus vulnerability endorsed by technicolour film and high production values.

Although ostensibly offering a critique of nurse training and the harsh restrictions on student nurses, the vocational ideal is heavily emphasised. A stance on nursing issues is clearly articulated by the Matron at several points in both films: that the deep happiness to be found in nursing is that of being of service. The book on which *The Feminine Touch* is based, *A Lamp is Heavy* by Sheila Mackay Russell, is critical of precisely this attitude, but the film is infused with a self-sacrificing ethos. This is undoubtedly due to the influence of the film's nursing adviser, the Matron of a famous London teaching hospital, and screenwriter Monica Dickens. Dickens seems to see no incongruities in this move to a more romanticised and sentimental view of nursing life in spite of her earlier critique of nursing as 'boring drudgery' in her autobiographical novel *One Pair of Feet*.

The only film that treats nursing work with the kind of matter-of-factness with which doctoring is treated throughout this period is, rather surprisingly, a low budget comedy and minor 'B' movie screen filler, *Twice Round the Daffodils* (GB 1962). Made in black and white on what was clearly a minimal budget, this story of life in a TB sanatorium focuses on a men's ward in the care of Catty, a nurse who is shown to be more than capable of coping with her difficult patients, in both physical and psychological terms. Although tending towards the 'ministering angel' stereotype, Catty is neither a prudish asexualised virgin nor a doctor's handmaiden. The nurses are shown to have a considerable degree of autonomy, only falling under the jurisdiction of a rather distant Matron. As well as coping with routine nursing tasks, they have to deal with the psychological problems created by long-term illness and hospital confinement, including anger, depression and sexual frustration; no doctors are depicted, although there are veiled references to their presence.

Against this positive image, nurses in this film are set up as sexual spectacles for male voyeuristic pleasure. At one point, a nurse loses her skirt, 'unknowingly' revealing a classic voyeuristic fantasy of frilly knickers, suspenders and stockings to the male patients hiding voyeuristically in the cupboard – and, of course, the film audience.[31] The nurse revealed on the screen is not just a '*Carry On*' joke, but the depiction of a fantasy which gained increasing visibility during the 1960s as women's clothes were removed on the screen to attract the male audience back to the cinema. Competition from a new leisure rival, television, led to demands from the film industry for a relaxation of censorship. Nurses suffered the same fate as other female characters, revealing shapely sexualised bodies beneath fetishistic uniforms. Catty, as a ministering angel, manages to avoid this fate but predictably, by the closing frames of the film, she is engaged to one of her patients.

Fascination and aspiration: the romantic ideal

From the mid-1950s to the mid-1960s, an unusually high number of films were produced which used a hospital environment as their background. Most of these films featured doctors in leading roles, but there were also a substantial number of films which in some way profiled nursing. Medicine and nursing began to feature heavily in other popular genres, particularly in the romantic fictions of Mills & Boon, publishers specialising in the production of cheap, mass-produced paperbacks for a primarily female readership. In the cultural analysis of popular fiction production, considerable attention has been paid to the concept of romance and how romance operates as pornography for women (Snitow 1984). Given the general attitude of critical disparagement towards this form of popular literature and its readership, feminists have been concerned with finding in the activity of reading a recuperative impulse, one that can be analysed as some form of resistance to dominant (patriarchal and capitalist) values. Several studies have attempted to examine the relationship between female desire, pleasure and romantic fiction, most notably perhaps Tania Modleski's *Loving with a Vengeance* (1984) and *Reading the Romance* by Janice Radway (1984). The approach I use focuses on the underlying ideological assumptions of the texts, the ideas and images that writers – all of them women, many of them trained as nurses – were drawing on to engage their readers, rather than the activity of reading itself.

Two of the women I interviewed claimed that an aspiration to become middle-class attracted them to nursing, rather than romantic fantasy; the same motivations, coupled with a fascination for medical knowledge, can compel the reading of medical romances. In her analysis of the 1950s audience for medical programmes on television such as *Your Life in Their Hands* (BBC 1958–64) Karpf points out that female viewers by and large formed the majority of the audience. Most of the programmes at this time belong to a category that she labels 'the medical approach' which sees the history of medicine as a triumphant narrative, 'a soaring graph of progress, with successive scientific discoveries and breakthroughs extending human knowledge and curative powers, and replacing primitive nostrums and folk remedies' (Karpf 1988a: 111). In the late 1950s the 'medical approach' to sickness and disease was at its peak in Britain, unchallenged by the consumerist lobby that grew throughout the 1960s along with other powerful resistance and liberation movements. Nor was it challenged by a 'look after yourself' approach which began to percolate into government health policy in the early 1950s as the result of a growing recognition of the cost of providing free at point of delivery health care services. Throughout the 1950s, the medical establishment was at the summit of popular belief in its power to cure and heal, with the result that doctors became folk heroes in popular stories, replacing sons of the gentry and other minor aristocrats as symbols of masculine power and virility.

The very concept of romance as a way of arranging reproduction between women and men is peculiarly Western. Bridget Fowler points out that the material conditions for romance as a 'structure of feeling' are first of all agrarian capitalism, and secondly, the patriarchal mode of domestic production (Fowler 1991: 19). The pre-conditions for romantic literature as a genre are a fusion of the classic realist narrative form of the nineteenth-century novel with that of an older form, the fairy or folk tale. Modleski locates the sentimental novel as a precursor to Harlequin romances, a lineage that she traces back through the novels of Charlotte Brontë and Jane Austen. In the classic (sentimental novel) formula, 'the heroine, who is often of lower social status than the hero, holds out against his attacks on her "virtue" until he sees no other recourse than to marry her. Of course, by this time he wants to marry her, having become smitten with her sheer "goodness" (Modleski 1984: 17). This structure underlies the formula of most doctor/nurse romances in the 1950s.

In her exploration of the romance genre in 1930s magazines, Fowler points to the frequency of the Madonna/whore dyad, where the Madonna has a 'consuming commitment to duty', self-sacrifice (usually defined as love), and 'displays her work ethic within the family as an extension of this duty to the other' (Fowler 1991: 57). Images of 'the industrious wife' who provides personal services for her husband in the form of domestic labour replace the philanthropic ideal of the (Victorian) middle-class wife who occupies herself with good causes; virtue is exemplified through pre-marital and extra-marital chastity. The heroes of these stories are mainly businessmen and their sons, with doctors running a close second. According to Fowler, the doctor is the chivalric knight (of the Proppian fairy tale[32]), and like him he must pass various tests and demolish numerous obstacles before being rewarded with romantic marriage; he has to prove himself not only a worthy suitor, but a morally superior male. The stories depict a commitment to professional values reigning supreme over other emotions (such as financial motivations or emotional entanglements); in order to prove himself worthy, the chivalric knight has a disinterested duty to kill but the doctor must disinterestedly save (Fowler 1984: 123). Elements of the moral and ethical interests of the nineteenth-century domestic novel with its roots in the Protestant work ethic are foregrounded in these stories, where the only 'villain' to be overcome is death itself.

Analysis of romantic novels has tended to concentrate on either the unconscious structure of romance (Pearce and Stacey 1995) or broader patterns and themes (Paizis 1998) rather than on studies of specific genres at particular times (Fowler's work is one of the few exceptions). The doctor/nurse romance is a very particular variation of the romance genre's format. Medical romances of one sort or another were popular in the 1930s, but it was only in the late 1950s that nurses became integral to the formula and that the books became widespread and popular, not only in Britain but also in North America. The reasons for this historical conjuncture are complex, and involve examining a matrix of factors drawn together here around two axes, female fascination and aspiration; before dealing with each in turn I want to situate these 'structures of feeling' within the broader framework of 1950s culture, social history and femininity.

Stepping back and taking a broader look at the position of women in 1950s and 1960s Britain, what becomes apparent is the contradictory attitudes to their role as workers and their domestic responsibilities as mothers. In her analysis of the position of married women and their relationship with the newly emergent welfare state, Elizabeth Wilson argues that most female commentators and activists of the time considered the cause of 'reasonable' feminism to have been won. Women had gained the right to vote, to education, and had access of some sort to most careers; during the 1950s they won, in theory, the right to equal pay in the civil service and in teaching. Popular magazines of the day such as *Woman* and *Woman's Own* are filled with images of the 'New Woman' happily doing the housework with her new labour-saving devices; but hidden behind the painted smiles of the 1950s housewife there lurked a darker picture. Throughout the period, the number of women in the workforce actually increased from 21 per cent in 1951 to 32 per cent by 1961 (Westergaard and Resler (1975) quoted in Wilson 1980: 41). On the one hand women were inveigled by popular magazines and TV programmes to believe that their place was in the home; they were presented with recipes for dinner parties, sewing projects, household hints and decorating tips. Advertisers taunted women, trying to persuade them that domestic drudgery could be fun and pleasure if they bought the latest labour-saving devices. But the catch-22 for many women was that to be able to afford the latest domestic appliance they had to go out to work; it was a period of economic boom and jobs were plentiful. Women were vociferously told in publications and texts of all kinds that their place was in the home, yet they were also persuaded that they had to work for the financial benefit of the family. In one of the few books on the subject written at the time, *Women's Two Roles: Home and Work*, Viola Klein and Alva Myrdal try to assess the impact of these conflicting demands on women's lives, but find little evidence of any systematic research into the problem (Wilson 1980).

Wendy Webster argues that the role of indigenous women as primarily wives and mothers was facilitated by the recruitment of women from (former) colonial territories such as Africa and the Caribbean to work in low paid public sector service jobs (1998: xi). The women and men who arrived in Britain to work found a cold welcome awaiting them. Black women were expected to work cleaning hospitals, offices, hotels, public toilets and the London Underground, work that was not only menial and demeaning but seen as suitable because it was 'dirty'. Evelyn Nakano Glenn argues that the racial division of paid labour in the United States shifted from the private to the public sphere between the wars, with black women employed to do menial 'back room' chores such as cooking and cleaning and caring for the sick elderly in nursing homes and hospitals, work that kept them invisible. In the same settings, 'White women are disproportionately employed as lower level professionals (e.g. nurses and social workers), technicians and administrative support workers to carry out the more skilled and supervisory tasks' (Glenn 1992: 20). A similar situation developed in Britain in the 1950s: black workers were denied opportunities to work in shops, in clerical jobs or in the restaurant sector; there was a resistance to employing black labour 'in jobs that involved "contact with the public"' (Patterson 1963: 101, quoted in Webster 1998: 159). Many of those who came to Britain left their homes in the hope of finding a better life for themselves and their families but were met by signs advertising accommodation that stated 'no coloureds, no Irish'. Forced into the furnished private rental sector where the facilities such as bathrooms, sinks and hot water were woefully inadequate, black people were considered to be 'dirty' and 'primitive' because of overcrowded living conditions produced through racism (Webster 1998: 175). Irrespective of differences in skills, occupations and ethnicities black people were constructed as 'all of the same kind'; many who were teachers, for example, were not given jobs in spite of the shortage of trained staff and became downwardly mobile.[33] Black women, constructed as 'workers', were not wanted as mothers and denied many of the benefits of the expanded post-war welfare state such as housing and nursery provision (Webster 1998).

The attitudes of the era are scattered across a range of films and television programmes. Lola Young has systematically analysed the few films made by white filmmakers in the 1950s and 1960s that articulate inter-racial tensions, arguing that many of the problems are depicted as specifically sexual (Young 1996). Eugenicist arguments that black people had 'measurable and largely inheritable, physical attributes below the average for the United Kingdom' still held currency in the 1950s (Bertram 1958: 21, quoted in Young 1996: 87). Fears of black people were voiced in terms of a threatening fecundity, of 'over-running' the country with a source of cheap labour; this imaginary threat to the white working-class finds its clearest expression on television in *Till Death Us Do Part* which began in 1966 and was watched by eighteen million viewers.[34] Warren Mitchell played the infamous foul-mouthed bigot Alf Garnett who gave vent to a tirade of reactionary prejudices, xenophobia and hypocrisy. In a review in the *London Evening Standard* in 1968, Milton Shulman refers to Garnett as a monstrous social aberration that, 'like some boil on the back of the neck that one cannot resist stroking or touching', demands the nation's attention (Daniels and Gerson 1989: 27).

Formations of black femininity were largely invisible apart from in popular culture where black women were constructed as exotically sexual; formations of white femininity continued to emphasise duty and sacrifice as women's true nature, although the picture was often contradictory. On the one hand, there appeared to be more opportunities for women than ever before; on the other, women who opted for a career in a traditional profession like nursing often did so because of the lack of other opportunities available, particularly for lower middle- and working-class women. It was still extremely difficult for a woman to get into medical school unless 'daddy was a doctor', and even then she had to have higher qualifications than her male peers. Educated women tended to enter the other great female profession, teaching, where nationalisation of the education system had created a demand for teachers analogous to that in nursing. The only other obvious options for women with a modicum of education were secretarial work and banking, a situation that continued virtually unchanged until the mid-1970s. Whatever work a woman chose to do, however, it was expected that she would give it up, if not when she married, then when the children were born. For many men with middle-class aspirations working in clerical jobs in the emerging retail and service sectors – such as my father – having a non-working wife was a symbol of their upwardly mobile success and their ability to provide the family with the new products of affluence. In this scenario, the woman's role was to manage the household and tend the home – this was an era when traditionally 'feminine' crafts such as needlework, knitting and cookery dominated much of popular non-fiction literature written by and for women.

The increasing popularity of romantic fiction throughout this period is, in part, a reflection of women's increasing literacy. The 1944 Education

Act had ensured that all children had the statutory right to education, initially to the age of 14, then 15 and later 16. The debate about what kind of education girls should have was frustrated by a lack of statistical data, but by the early 1960s it was apparent that the overall proportion of girls to boys staying on at school had not increased. The assumption was that once girls married their education would be wasted; this was particularly true of official attitudes towards working-class girls. The Crowther Report (1959) states that 'the prospect of courtship and marriage should rightly influence the education of the adolescent girl' (Baker 1989: 11), and the Newsom Report four years later (1963) reiterated the same sentiments, claiming that girls should be learning feminine skills. In spite of this gloomy picture of the prospects for women of gaining a university place, all women were educated to the age of 15, and more women were passing the eleven plus examination for secondary education at a grammar (academic) school than boys. It therefore seems probable that the overall literacy level of the female population was rising throughout this period (Baker 1989: 12). This was certainly the view of the publishers responsible for the mass production of gothic romances in early 1960s America. Reaching white middle-class women and retaining them as a reading public who would regularly consume their products was one of the reasons that this particular genre became so successful (Radway 1984: 32).

But there were other influences on people's lives that signalled a major change for many white women in terms of their collective experience. Much has been made in histories of the cinema and television at this time of the move away from urban centres to the suburbs. In the post-war period, inner city housing stock in Britain was in a deplorable state as a result of neglect by landlords and bombing raids during the war. New building commenced on the peripheries of major conurbations as part of the new state welfare policies, resulting in a rash of 'new towns' such as Kirkby on the outskirts of Liverpool which was built to house the inhabitants of one of the poorest inner city areas. People were removed from the communities in which their families had lived for several generations, breaking up the pattern of life and placing them, often in isolation, on the new estates. People were encouraged to own their homes and mortgages were made easier for the ordinary working man (not women) to obtain; house building boomed as more and more people moved to the new estates in the suburbs. A change in patterns of leisure activities developed as a result – gardening, 'do it yourself' and television viewing all became popular. For the women targeted as consumers by TV advertising and popular magazines – mainly the wives of upper working-class ('blue collar') and lower middle-class ('white collar') men reaping the benefits of the 1950s economic boom and apparent affluence – the benefits of all this were mixed. For those fortunate enough to possess them, the new modern houses and domestic appliances certainly lightened the domestic workload, but isolation from female relatives and friends increased the burden of childcare and reduced opportunities for 'letting off steam' (Wilson 1980).

Reading books and magazines and watching television were popular leisure pursuits for women isolated at home, a situation exploited keenly by book publishers. In a press release written in 1988 to celebrate eighty years in publishing, Mills & Boon explain their perception of the relationship between the new consumer culture, reading romances and watching television:

> In the 1950s the editorial style of Mills & Boon swung away from the harsh realities of the previous decade, and took on a fairy-tale quality; stories were exotic, taking readers away from Britain and the memory of war with international travel, foreign names and places. Colourful detail became still more important, and covers featured holiday resorts, dance halls and pretty dresses. Towards the late 1950s, however, lending libraries began to decline, and with them, Mills & Boon's major outlet. Readers could not afford hardback books, romance paperbacks were not yet available, and the taste for romantic fiction itself had not waned. It was the arrival of television, originally feared to be the downfall of reading, that provided the solution. The Doctor/Nurse theme, already successful for Mills & Boon, became suddenly more popular via television medical dramas. In response to this vogue, a small paperback publishing firm in Canada, Harlequin, approached Mills & Boon for the North American rights to some of the Doctor/Nurse titles, to then be produced under the Harlequin imprint. So successful was this enterprise that in 1960, Mills & Boon was able to turn its attention to the launching of its own paperback series.
>
> (Mills & Boon, untitled press release, 1988)

According to the publishers, it was the popularity of medical melodramas and medical romances that fuelled the transition in Britain from hardback to paperback novels, and Mills & Boon's expansion into the North American market. The rise in popularity of this particular form of the romance articulates a change in feminine values which was to have a particular resonance in public attitudes towards nurses.

While it has become unpopular to speculate about the activity of reading without empirical and ethnographic work, I intend to contemplate the appeal of doctor/nurse romances despite the dearth of empirical material available on the subject. First of all, the sample; it consists of more than forty Mills & Boon romances published between 1957 and 1989, clearly a very small number in relation to the overall numbers produced (some four a month since the early 1960s). Out of these, I have concentrated on those featuring hospital nurses at the centre of the narrative, with an emphasis on books about nurse training. Amongst the earlier books I have managed to obtain, a significant number concentrate on the experiences of initiates. Interestingly, three authors dominate these earlier texts, all of whom have a detailed knowledge of hospital life and medical and nursing procedures. There is a clear demarcation between those authors who use the hospital as a background for a romantic drama, and those who include the hospital setting as part of the drama. For example, *Staff Nurse* (Valerie Nelson 1957) is a romance written in the style of the sentimental novel, with issues of class, social etiquette, breeding and money heavily foregrounded in the plot. In contrast, *Junior Pro* (Kate Norway 1959) is far more concerned with the contemporary conflict between marriage and career and the relationship between work and femininity. Whereas *Staff Nurse* promotes a religious, vocational picture of nursing with self-sacrifice, self-abasement and self-abnegation as the ideals encapsulated by the heroine, it nonetheless constantly states a preference for marriage, claiming that 'helping and encouraging a man in his career is the finest work a woman can do' (Nelson 1957: 127). In this view of nursing, the job is a stepping stone towards a well-bred marriage, and career nurses are viewed as deviant women. In many of the books, what is established is not a problem with women working as nurses *per se*, but a view of career nurses (women in authority) as hard and masculinised. These women are always single, never partnered with anyone, appearing alone and friendless; there is no hint of lesbian activity and/or relationships. In *Junior Pro*, nurses remain single not so much out of dedication to their work but because the work leaves them no energy for being social (Norway 1959: 107). Although this narrative follows all the conventions of the stock romantic plot (older man, younger woman, two suitors and a scene where the heroine removes her clothes out of contingency thus 'innocently' arousing the passions of her admirer), the heroine insists on completing her training and obtaining her qualifications before she marries. The narrative resolution to this commitment to work is posed in terms of a 1950s notion of middle-class marriage which promotes separate but equal spheres of responsibility. The nurse and her doctor husband will be 'one person doing one job' (Norway 1959: 157).

Amongst nursing heroines of this period, a surprisingly high number come from the country, from farms, villages and small country towns. The hospital tends to be situated in the city, a juxtaposition which has particular resonance in literature. The country tends to be metonymic for values associated with goodness, honesty, order, 'the natural', the city with corruption, insincerity and disorder and 'the cultural'. Within the city, the hospital operates as a large country house, a repository of the diminishing aristocratic values of the country. Hierarchy and order are maintained through traditional class and gender divisions. Threats to this order come in the form of 'outsiders': for example, in *The Lambs* (Kate Norway 1965) a

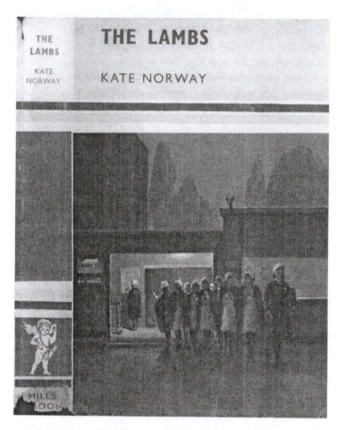

Figure 2.4 Cover, *The Lambs*, Kate Norway (Mills & Boon®, 1965)

young woman is accepted for nurse training who is on probation. A debate ensues about whether this 'type' of girl is·suitable to be a nurse. Most of the nursing heroines are recognisably middle-class and white, with few exceptions. Where black nurses are featured, they are also middle-class, their parents' occupations specifically stated. Black nurses in these stories are always 'one of our [white] kind', alone and dependent on white cultural values. In *Night Duty at Dukes*, the Jamaican nurse Theo discusses her marriage prospects with a friend, concluding, 'I don't want to go home and marry one of my own people. I've come to like Englishmen better. That's an awful thing to say, isn't it?' (Bess Norton 1960, Corgi edition 1974: 29).

Southern Englishness is given a primary value in these stories – Welshness and Northernness are given deviant, superstitious values that obstruct the rationality of modern medicine. Foreignness is seen as threatening and disturbing, strange, unknowable and therefore ultimately untrustworthy.[35]

Given that these entrenched ideological values and attitudes underlie a great many of the stories, it is perhaps surprising to find that the one thing that they unequivocally share is support for the NHS. In numerous stories, private patients' privileges are seen as unfair and unjustified: 'Just because they've got money, why on earth should they expect to be treated as though their lives were more valuable than anyone else's?' (*The Lambs* 1965: 79). Dedication to medicine for the sake of suffering humanity is given positive value, practising medicine as a way of making money or conferring social status viewed negatively. Nurses in these stories always marry doctors who support the positive values, so that in giving up their public role to support their doctor husbands, they are continuing to support the ideals and beliefs that have informed them as nurses. Their power as women becomes the power of social influence, and it is perhaps here that the attraction lies for the reader. To have money, social status and influence without compromising personal ideas or beliefs was certainly my mother's fantasy as an upwardly mobile post-war wife and mother, a fantasy that Carolyn Steedman claims has not been recognised or become visible because it stands outside the academic discourses that theorise working-class women's experience (Steedman 1986).

Aspiration cannot be wholly separated from the other strong attraction exerted by these texts, a fascination with medical knowledge and power. In some texts, knowledge and power is encapsulated in the figure of the brilliant surgeon whose new surgical procedures will save people from death. The doctor tends to remain a distant, unknown figure whose 'truth' is discovered by the heroine once she decides to trust him. In some texts doctors are more humane characters; the mysteries of medical science are revealed to them and the nursing heroines through the narrative, involving the reader in solving medical mysteries and health problems. In initiate stories in particular, readers learn with new nursing recruits the language of medicine, including terminologies for describing the body and its functions and the shorthand or slang of hospital communication. The reader learns something of medical discourse, as well as the power relations that are built into that discourse. These books offer the pleasure of 'insider' knowledge of hospital life, without having to be involved in the hard and dirty work of nursing – a point emphasised on the first page of *Junior Pro* where nursing is described as hard work, 'not a thing you learn from books' (Norway 1959: 1).

The doctor/nurse romances of the late 1950s and early 1960s amalgamate fantasies of white middle-class lifestyle with illusions of medical knowledge and power into a single generic form, satisfying a demand for stories in which female characters gain access to social status, power and knowledge through trading on the cultural capital of their sexuality and femininity. Although the books ostensibly support an ethos of white, middle-class patriarchal authority in the form of their doctor heroes, that ethos is

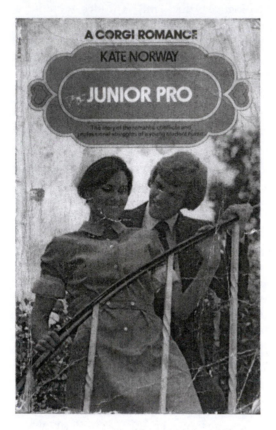

Figure 2.5 Cover, *Junior Pro*, Kate Norway (Corgi, 1974; first published by Mills & Boon®, 1959)

nonetheless shown to be flawed: men who represent both curing and caring for the common good are shown to be relatively rare, with doctors more commonly depicted as 'villainous' for selling their services privately. This ethical and moral standpoint reworks paternalistic liberal humanist values into a welfare statist framework of commitment to equality of care, but leaves traditional class distinctions relatively intact through the advocacy of professionalism. By giving the hospital the ethos of a large country house, gender roles also remain undisturbed. The frequent references to Florence Nightingale and the descriptions of nursing work tend towards what Poovey (1989) has termed 'housewifeliness'. Nonetheless, the texts are critical of certain masculinist assumptions about women's work as nurses, often stressing how nurses, as mediators between the patient and the doctor, play a crucial role in both the saving of lives and the promotion of patient well-being. In many of the texts, the picture is one of nurses as a competent and capable group of women who quite often do the thinking for men, but never take the credit for it. Their sexual desires, described as actively seeking satisfaction through pleasure in kissing and touching, become sublimated through 'good' doctors into a quasi-religious ecstasy centred on the male because he will do 'good' in the world. The welling emotions and tears aroused by the texts are cathartic in the sense of releasing the pent-up feelings and emotions that unfulfilled expectancies and promises in everyday life generate. As one nurse who reads these romances commented, they speak to desires for a medical utopia that she feels she still needs to cling to.

Soap, sex and satire: the late 1960s and early 1970s

The 1960s in British society are now seen by some as a time of turbulence and unrest, a period when traditional class distinctions were overturned and there was a new sexual freedom. A more pessimistic view would regard many of these apparent changes as superficial; the deeper structures of British society were left relatively unchallenged and unchanged.

Throughout the 1950s, the growing impact of television and television's portrayal of medicine and nursing significantly contributed to public perceptions of and attitudes towards the two professions. In particular, two programmes in the late 1950s scored high on television audience rating scales: *Your Life in Their Hands* (BBC 1958–64), a documentary series that celebrated surgical intervention, high-technology curative medicine and pharmaceutical therapeutics; and the long-running *Emergency Ward 10* (ITV 1957–67), described at the time as a 'documentary drama' of hospital life, that focused on life-threatening conditions and heroic medical intervention. Between them, these two programmes changed the face of medical broadcasting in 1950s Britain from a preventative orientation to a curative one erasing 'all recollection of the fitness and fibre obsession from producers' minds' (Karpf 1988a: 50). No longer were medical broadcasters extolling listeners to take care of themselves and eat plenty of healthy foods; instead, viewers were to be informed and educated (and undoubtedly entertained) by the spectacle of modern surgical methods and procedures, with their accompanying narratives of successful intervention and cure.

Karpf sees this change in broadcasting practice, from the 'look after yourself approach' to the medical perspective, as part of a more generalised scientific enthusiasm pervading 1950s society. To paraphrase her, the 1950s bubbled with therapeutic optimism; it was the era of Sputnik, of the development of space technology, which seemed to exemplify the Macmillan government's 'you've never had it so good' conservative credo. The new 'age of affluence' had an unbounded belief in the potential and efficacy of science and technology; chemicals and pharmaceutical manufacturing led the field in the creation of new industrial complexes (and empires). Along with economic expansion and a growing market for goods and services came notions of consumer choice. Instead of being addressed as an aggregated mass, the public were increasingly hailed as consumers and individuals. By early 1961, a pamphlet accompanying the series *Your Life in Their Hands* talked of the importance of medical research and the value of medical scientific methods, reflecting a growing belief in research as a panacea and doctors as a 'superior race of human beings whose calling raises them from the ordinary level of human fellowship' (Karpf 1988a: 52–3). This phase of programming marked the beginning of what Karpf refers to as an infatuation with the London teaching hospitals – an infatuation that is also clearly apparent in films like *The Feminine Touch* (1956) and much of the popular doctor/nurse romantic literature of the time.

Karpf stresses that by the beginning of the second series of *Your Life in Their Hands*, television's imperatives for drama and excitement had begun to play a major role in the shaping of these documentary programmes. New technology using videotape recording (available for the first time in 1956) was enabling coverage of the operating table to be far more intimate. The television audience had grown markedly throughout the 1950s, a growth reflected in the purchase of TV licences, from 343,000 in 1950 to 10 million by 1960 (Docherty, Morrison and Tracey 1987: 23). Independent television had effectively challenged the BBC's monopoly, to the extent that the BBC had a new constituency, its audience, whose needs had to be taken care of. While the BBC were intent on conveying the 'liveness' and excitement of real-life medical dramas, the producer of ATV's *Emergency Ward 10* (ITV 1957–67) had a slightly different agenda; 'We wanted to overcome the pre-war attitude of the British public to hospitals as institutions, places to be avoided at all costs. We wanted people to respond to new research in medicine' (quoted in Karpf 1988a: 183). Like many of its counterparts in medical romantic fiction, *Emergency Ward 10* was characterised by plots that dealt with life and death crises and rare infectious diseases; it used a great deal of medical jargon and portrayed doctors as 'boisterous young philanderers with an unquestionable sense of vocation' (Karpf, *ibid.*).

Only two of the later episodes of this long-running series are available for viewing in the National Film Archive; much of the series was transmitted live and never recorded on film or videotape, but from this rather limited source it is possible to get a sense of the programme. Perhaps most striking to a contemporary viewer is its static visual field; there is only the slightest suggestion of a ward (and a world) beyond the bedside, where most of the action takes place. The drama is script-led, with the cameras following the doctors, who do most of the talking and motivate the action. When nurses speak in a doctor's presence, which is usually to ask a question or clarify a suggested course of treatment, the camera rarely cuts to them. Nurses are background characters who take orders and occasionally explain medical dialogue to patients, acting as a conduit for information and as translators of medical terminology for the viewer. Class relations between doctors, nurses and patients are explicitly referred to in the dialogue; working-class patients refer to the doctors as 'stuck up'. Amongst the nurses, there is some slight variation in accent, but little to differentiate them otherwise. Nurses obey doctors' orders without question on the wards, although there is one scene in which a nurse queries a doctor's diagnosis of her own medical condition. Nonetheless, the overall picture is one of male medical control. The doctors are all white, male and middle-class, and it is they who control the fictional diegesis through their use of medical discourse. The patients in these particular episodes are working-class in most cases except for one woman, cast as an Asian immigrant, who is the focus of medical concern. She remains virtually speechless throughout the examination, an object of the medical gaze mediated by the camera. In the doctors' dialogue, her 'otherness' is seen as the cause of their mis-diagnosis: 'The colour of her skin foxed us at first. Like clots, we thought the pigmentation inside her mouth was normal for her.' Her helplessness is a function of a realist aesthetic that attempts to incorporate social issues into the body of the text – a text that presents the healthy white, male middle-class body as the 'norm' against which other bodies are compared.[36] In this world view, disease and ill health are the property and problems of 'others' – women, the working class, the impaired and non-whites.

Throughout its ten-year run, *Emergency Ward 10* received praise for its attention to accuracy of medical detail, but became increasingly criticised for its focus on the personal lives of the medical staff. Press reviews reveal that the programme made some attempt to deal with contemporary issues in the health service, portraying an unauthorised meeting of nurses to discuss a pay claim (May 1962), a nurse getting sacked (December 1963), and a love affair between a white house surgeon and his black female colleague (July 1964), parts of which were banned by the Independent Television Authority (ITA) because they were considered 'too suggestive'. The *Daily Telegraph* loudly proclaimed that these cuts 'had nothing to do with colour prejudice at all' (17/7/64) but given that a racialised discourse of 'miscegenation' continued to permeate heterosexual relations between black and white couples, the claim has a hollow ring.[37] By 1965 the success of the drama in dealing with medically related social issues and promoting health education campaigns was acknowledged by the Ministry of Health, although how they reached this conclusion is unclear. The series faded out in 1967 largely unremarked, no doubt because of the increasing presence of American medical dramas with their own particular blend of high production values and handsome young doctors accompanied by pretty young nurses in short-skirted sexy uniforms. In their extensive analysis of American TV's image of nursing, Kalisch and Kalisch point out that throughout this period the nurse is a silent handmaiden who does little identifiable nursing work (Kalisch and Kalisch 1982a). Even her role of patient advocate and mediator is taken over by sympathetic medical men.

Given the preference shown by the audience in the mid- and late 1960s for the compassionate, caring American medic, whether he is Dr Kildare, Ben Casey or Marcus Welby, it is worth speculating why nurses disappear into romantic fictions and doctors dominate small screen melodramas. Karpf sees these dramas reaching beyond the conventions of the human interest story to endorse expression of feelings such as vulnerability and fear, emotions more commonly articulated by women. The doctor in these stories is often a wise man who mediates family relationships and restores harmony. In a decade marked by the opening up of difference between men and women, black and white, left and right, 'the doctor programmes reasserted hope and social stability, healing the damage and offering reassurance that the system could succour and patriarchy provide' (Karpf 1988a: 191). Karpf's speculations may be on the right lines, but it is worth noting some of the reasons why these dramas were so successful on American TV. In an in-depth analysis of the relationship between television and medical power, Joseph Turow (1989) points out that the formula for medical melodramas has remained largely unchanged since *Dr Kildare* was first serialised on the cinema screen in the 1930s. In 1961, an enterprising producer tried to break with the formulaic pattern of the Kildare/Ben Casey format by developing a series that was based entirely on nurses. *The Nurses* ran for three series over three years, but from the early days it was predicted that a reliance on female leading characters would eventually be the cause of the show's downfall because there were no heroic males to attract male viewers during prime-time viewing. While this argument may seem a little surprising – the audience for medical melodrama has, in Britain at least, been conceived as primarily female – when it is placed in the context of American network programming policy at this time, it makes more sense. Programme production was not targeted to appeal to specific groups of people, but operated on the principle of common denominator factors; the audience for every show had to be maximised, and high ratings were the only criteria for success. Since male viewers at this time tended to control prime-time evening viewing (from 7 pm to 10 pm) shows mixed action and melodrama in an effort to appeal to both sexes. Advertisers were less interested in shows that dealt with social and ethical issues, more interested in those that entertained people. This led to a number of policy changes in the screening of medical melodramas which were nails in the coffin for *The Nurses*. Medical series had to be screened in the late evening, the shows had to revolve around male physicians and the dramas had to enact highly emotional issues of life and death, not the politics of the hospital or the medical system (Turow 1989). The changes in programming policy, instituted throughout American network television, ended what Kalisch and Kalisch consider to be one of the most positive representations of nurses to appear on the small screen (Kalisch and Kalisch 1982a). It is worth noting, though, that *The Nurses* did not please American nurses at the time, most of whom vented their criticism via their professional associations and the nursing journals (Turow 1989).

The Nurses was never shown in Britain. Throughout the 1960s, American medical melodrama imports such as *Dr Kildare* entertained the British television audience with high-tech life and death drama, where nurses featured as background presences or occasionally as efficient personal assistants for the doctor heroes; any sense of personal autonomy or professionalism was completely absent. These shows attracted large audiences during primetime, no doubt reflecting their attraction for the male as well as the female viewer since it seems likely, based on later research evidence, that male household members controlled later evening viewing (Morley 1986, 1992). The combination of machismo and melo in these shows clearly reworks 1950s ideas about nursing as a vocation that serves its own ideology of care into a 1960s ethos of self-abnegating servility to medicine, rendering fictional nurses virtually silent, visible only as decoration and sexual spectacle.

If nurses were invisible as active agents on the small screen, on the large screen they continued to be sexualised objects of scorn and derision. In British films, nurses are figures of fun, albeit with less clothing on than in the previous decade; the *Carry On* series and the *Doctor* films keep on lampooning them throughout the 1960s. In many foreign films, they became creatures of sex. Following the general drift in American films of this period towards misogynistic images of women, nurses became devious criminals (*The Burning Court* US 1963, *Nurse-Made* US 1970), murderers (*The Honeymoon Killers* US 1970), prostitutes (*Woman of Desire* US 1968) and nymphomaniacs (*I, A Woman* Den. 1966) or they are the subjects of violence: they get murdered (*Night of Bloody Horror* US 1969, *The Strangler* US 1964), raped (*Day-Dream* Jap 1964) and generally abused (*Temptation* US 1962). Most of these pictures date from after 1962, the point at which the Hays (Production) Code, regulator of Hollywood's moral conduct, was defeated by an action in the Supreme Court ending a system of censorship which had remained virtually unchanged since 1934 (Randall 1977, Maltby 1983). The image of nurses as sex objects has not been dealt with in any depth in any of the existent literature on the nursing image. Nurses have been constructed as whores and prostitutes since Victorian times, but this image has been heavily policed by social mores with more or less help from the censor depending on the overall social climate. The professional view seems to be that it is better ignored, rather than discussed and aired. This silence still meets those who try to open up debate on the subject, as I discovered in my initial attempts to research it.

One British film, more than any other, seems to sum up fictional representations of nursing and hospitals on the small and large screen by the early 1970s. Released hot on the heels of *Carry On Matron* (GB 1972),

The National Health or Nurse Norton's Affair (GB 1973) mixes tragedy and farce in a satirical comedy that mocks Britain's ailing NHS, situating the action in contemporary Britain and its troubled economic climate. The film opens with a shot of a pillared portico hospital entrance and the sound of a public address system (PA) exhorting the hospital staff to use less hot water because the boiler is failing. The country house style architecture may call to mind nostalgic memories of a great and noble past, but the soundtrack contradicts any notion of an idealised or romantic view of the present. Cutting to an internal shot, an Afro-Caribbean nurse in tradi-tional uniform escorts a white male patient down a corridor where an Asian woman wearing a sari is on her knees scrubbing the floor. Entering the ward, a general air of anarchy prevails; a patient tears around in a wheel-chair and the male patients cat-call abuse at the nurses who try to smile cheerfully through the chaos. In the kitchen, the porters sit smoking and drinking tea while the PA calls in vain for Dr Singh. In the patients' sitting room an American medical melodrama, 'Nurse Norton's Affair', is just beginning on the television. The opening shots emphasise the modern hospital, its wide corridors, comfortable patient rooms and high-tech medical support systems; the contrast with the ailing British NHS hospital is immediate and obvious, but as the frozen images of the actors of the TV drama appear on the screen in the credit sequence, it becomes apparent that the tired, frazzled British nurses and doctors we have just seen are the stars of this glossy American series. The film cuts between these two fictional worlds, juxtaposing the ironically grim realism of British social issue drama with the high production values and melodramatic style of American prime-time television.

These contrasting styles show how the institutional and technological constraints of different production practices shape fictional realisms into specific representational forms. The black and white low budget soap format of *Emergency Ward 10* was superseded in the mid-1960s by American series melodramas with their glossy formats and high production values, a move that coincided with the introduction of colour TV viewing in Britain and the use of more aggressive advertising techniques by independent television. Additionally the mood and tone of the American product, with its emphasis on individual cure situations and the doctor as a heroic medical god, clearly suited the British medical discourse of 'cure' and its emphasis on research as the panacea that would solve the problems of ill health and disease. This discourse was prevalent in medical broadcasting because it met broadcast television's remit of educating and informing at a time when the BBC began to compete actively with ITV for viewers, adding spectacle as an entertaining ingredient to television producers' recipes for successful series in both fictional and documentary formats. Within the broadcasting envi-ronment, nursing's professional discourse of 'service' was taken at its word and nurses, as a group, did little to change the picture. This passive ethos began to be challenged in the late 1960s; for the first time, nurses began to complain vociferously about their outmoded working conditions, outdated pay scales and obsolete working practices. In the longer term this activist stance dramatically changed television's fictionalised stereotypes into a more complex and dynamic model.

The late 1960s and early 1970s were something of a watershed in nursing history, both in terms of the relationship between nursing and the NHS, and in terms of the internal battle for control of the profession between the Royal College of Nursing (RCN) and the nursing unions – principally the Confederation of Health Service Employees (COHSE) and the National Union of Public Employees (NUPE). In this fight for the hearts and minds of nurses, the media became a determining factor, establishing nurses' anger at their pay and conditions of work on the pages of every major daily newspaper and in many television news bulletins in a manner that has been barely equalled since.[38] The 'raise the roof' campaign (as it is now known in nursing history) was the first active involvement of the RCN with the media in a sustained campaign to pressurise the government to increase nurses' wages under a 'no-strike' banner. This was followed throughout the early 1970s by a series of trade union-led strike actions and workings to rule, which finally culminated in the nurses' pay settlement of 1974. What these pay disputes revealed was an underlying financial crisis – graphically ironised in *The National Health or Nurse Norton's Affair* – problems that would be brought into the living rooms of television viewers through the social realist format of the series *Angels* in a medical melodrama with a distinct difference. For the first time the focus was on nurses, their training and their work, encompassing both the detail of day-to-day nursing practice and, to a limited extent, the broader framework of operation circumscribed by limited resources and the dictates of NHS management policy. This series told the nurses' story for a change, leaving the medics on the periphery of the action.

First broadcast on BBC 1 in 1975, *Angels* was based on an idea by script editor Paula Milne, one of the first wave of female graduates from the National Film and Television School. It was written by female writers and produced by Julia Smith, latterly remembered for producing *Eastenders* and the failure of the BBC's early 1990s Euro soap *El Dorado*.[39] *Angels* quickly established itself as a popular favourite among young and old female viewers because of its strong female characters and positive portrayal of feminine values. So what was it about the series that was seen as different and how did it portray hospital life for working women?

In an article in *The Listener* (1975), Paula Milne claimed that the different approach to hospital drama taken by *Angels* was based on its series (rather than serial) format, with a team of writers independently responsible for each character rather than jointly developing storylines set against a hospital backdrop. In the early 1970s, serial drama was conventionally developed

by teams of writers who would generate storyline material against a background situation. This could equally be the hospital setting of, for example,
General Hospital (ATV 1972–9) or the motel setting of *Crossroads* (ATV
1964–88). Decisions on the detail of the storylines were made at script
conferences, a similar mode of production to that of American serial drama.
By changing the production format of *Angels* to a series, Milne changed
the narrative style, the way that information and pleasure are delivered to
the audience. This gave the programme a new 'authenticity' that was critically acclaimed for showing a more realistic view of nursing life. *Angels*
focused on the working lives of six student nurses at various stages in their
training – an approach somewhat analogous to the 'take four girls' approach
of the national recruitment drive for nurses current at that time. Each
writer was given a character to develop and required to research the specific
circumstances and situations that her character would encounter. This varied
from the experiences of young initiates coming into nursing straight from
school to the more experienced third year nurses who had served their
time on the wards. Only the first two of these early episodes of *Angels* are
available for viewing, so my commentary necessarily has a rather narrow
perspective. Nonetheless, it is obvious that *Angels* did not shirk from
refracting the nursing image through a critical prism, especially in its depiction of internal disputes concerning questions of authority between the
generations. It also addressed the thorny issue of pay and working conditions.

The opening sequences enact a masquerade of nursing identity that shows
the transformation from 'ordinary girl' to nurse through donning of the
distinctive uniform. This transformative sequence then cuts to the hospital
badge and the nursing image engraved upon it, a direct reference to
nursing's vocational roots in religious orders through the nun/nurse in her
habit and veil. The fictional hospital, St Angelas, is a representation of a
London teaching hospital with its ancient traditions in charitable care. The
choice is significant, enabling the producers to ignore the staffing shortages,
racial tensions and class issues raised by union activists working in the less
glamorous and poorer hospital sectors. By focusing on a high profile London
teaching hospital, *Angels* reinforces a particular professional ideal of nursing
at a time when the RCN's bid for hegemony was under severe stress due
to its stance on industrial action. Although this broader political framework
is engaged at the level of individual complaints and debates about pay
and conditions, the broader issues concerning the divided identity of the
profession were never addressed.

By concentrating on the experiences of six student nurses at different
stages in their training, *Angels* dramatised the experience of becoming a
nurse, showing how each individual negotiated the stresses and strains of
the training process. This approach emphasises the physically demanding
side of nursing work, not avoiding the 'dirty' aspects of patient care, the

irritatingly petty restrictions imposed by superiors, and the feelings of despondency and depression that most nurses have to deal with at some point or another during their training. The series dealt with conflict between nurses of different ages and rank as young initiates took on board increasing responsibilities and developed the skills and expertise necessary for final qualification. The initiates, representing particular feminine identities and differences, developed characterisations which took them beyond the simplistic stereotypes of nurses in, for example, *The Feminine Touch* (1956), but the programme's commitment to drama documentary now seems slowly staged and lacks in-depth analysis of the issues it was foregrounding. It did not investigate the deeper, structural changes in nursing that were occurring as a result of the instigation of the Salmon Report and re-organisation of the NHS in 1974.[40] By not addressing these institutional factors in more depth, *Angels* compromised, continuing to promote a feminine ideology of nursing at the very time that this ideology was beginning to be eroded.

Angels presents a middle-class drama of liberal individualism and ethical dilemmas in which national policy tends to be reduced to localised conflict between individuals. This is also true of the programme's depiction of racial conflict, which perpetuates a notion of racism as a personal problem of prejudiced individuals rather than a problem embedded in professional ideology and institutional culture. Compared with a later programme like *Casualty* (BBC 1 1985–date), which has foregrounded issues of policy, politics, 'race' and sexuality at different times, *Angels* now seems rather tame entertainment, a weak example of an issue-based drama. But it did alter the agenda for programme makers of medical drama by placing nurses at the centre of the action, and its high audience ratings (peaking at 12 million viewers) were a measure of its popularity and success.

Between the 1950s and the 1970s public perceptions of nurses changed markedly, a process mediated by the increasing presence on television of dramas and documentaries about medicine and hospital life. At the beginning of the 1950s, a strong service ethos pervaded notions of nursing identity and representation, an ethos implying that female nurses were held in high regard because they sacrifice notions of selfhood in order to serve others – primarily patients, but also the nursing profession itself. Nursing was regarded as hard and dirty work and a sense of vocation was considered essential in order to be able to do it. Throughout the 1950s and 1960s this image changed. No longer was nursing a noble profession (with an underlying implication of serving the nation): increasingly, nurses served medical ideologies of cure rather than nursing ideologies of care. Nowhere is this more apparent than in their servile relationships to the physical embodiment of these ideals, mythical god-like medical men. The development of independent television and the new international market in television programmes made images of the American doctor increasingly available to British audiences. Nurses became silent handmaidens in small screen melodramas, while on the big screen they were satirised as petty authoritarians and sexually frustrated 'battleaxes' or depicted as creatures of explicit sexuality. Only in the despised women's genre of romantic fiction could an image be found that gave nurses minds, bodies and voices of their own. Written by women for women, these stories told not only of passionate love between nurses and doctors, but negotiated a range of personal and moral issues around the meaning of nursing that began to appear in televisual form only after the nurses' pay campaigns challenged media representations of nursing as silent, self-sacrificing femininity. In these books, a fascination with medical men is part of a fascination with medical knowledge; to know one is to get to know the other, to see behind the mask of curative medicine to the driving (male) force behind it. The journey from innocence to experience that so many of these books portray is one that maps out the possibility of a career and marriage through partnership with a medical man. Caring is restored on an equal footing with curing because the man is dependent on the woman's capacity to provide it, and it is his acknowledgement of his need for her caring capacities that ultimately makes the nurse powerful.

By the late 1960s and early 1970s, nurses were actively altering public perceptions of their role through their campaigns for improved pay and better working conditions. The success of their claims raised their public profile, and sparked a new interest in the fictional representation of nursing, at least on television. *Angels* can certainly be seen as a product of a renewed level of public interest surrounding nurses and their role, but it is also a result of women in television making their mark by creating programmes centred on female characters. Submerged since the early 1950s into fantasies of male medical power and female subordination, the eruption of the nurse into speech and visibility in *Angels* coincided with the beginnings of what is now regarded as second wave feminism. Generally excluded from feminist accounts of the period because of its symbiotic relationship with femininity and the female caring role, nursing's stand against the state can nonetheless be seen as part of the general discontent with the low value given to women's role in society that swept through Britain during this period. The effects on the image of nursing can in retrospect be seen as significant; although *Angels* now looks dated because of its slow pace and visual style, for the first time a serious drama series was commissioned that totally centred on nurses. This was no small achievement for a female profession which throughout the post-war period had been either lampooned and satirised or, more commonly, completely ignored.

From the mid-1970s, nurses were increasingly aware of their image in the media, forming monitoring groups and pressure groups to try and maintain a sympathetic public consciousness of their role.[41] Over the years, this action has had limited success as more recent writings on nursing and the media point out (Salvage 1987a, Bridges 1990, Holloway 1992). Perhaps one reason for this is that nursing, while trying to present a united face to the public through its professional discourse of care, is in fact a deeply divided profession and has found it difficult to negotiate its differences in the rapidly changing health care environment of the latter years of the twentieth century. In the following chapter, these divisions are examined in some detail through an analysis of the research on recruitment and attrition, focusing on recruitment images and their relationship to nursing policy and practice.

3

THE PROFESSIONAL
IMAGINATION

Recruitment images share a symbiotic relationship with fictional images even though they appear to inhabit an ostensibly different discursive terrain. Fictional images circulate in spaces associated with leisure and consumption such as bookstalls and television series, recruitment images in careers and employment advice centres as well as leisure sites associated with advertising, such as magazines. Recruitment images have to communicate with their target groups so they use popular conceptions of nursing identity which they adapt or resist in various ways at different times. This chapter explores the dynamic between these two frameworks of nursing identity within the context of nursing's institutional and professional organisations and structures.

A divided identity

By the end of the nineteenth century, Nightingale's work had popularised nursing as an occupation for well-bred young ladies, many of whom were able to take up senior appointments in the major voluntary hospitals after a brief period of training. As this group became increasingly powerful, they were able to impose a stiff three-year training on new recruits and tried to prevent anyone who had not undergone this training from practising as a nurse (Vicinus 1985). In spite of Nightingale's opposition to a registration scheme that would, in effect, only recognise those who had undergone the three-year training as legitimate bearers of the title 'nurse', the professionalisers were eager to persuade the government that an Act of Registration was essential to safeguard both the public and the medical profession from unqualified practitioners.[1] The educational standards adopted for entry to training schemes were, however, too inflexible to produce enough nurses for all the kinds of nursing work that were needed. The poor in particular were rarely able to afford qualified nursing skills in their own homes, and the prestigious voluntary hospitals balked at the increased salary load they would have to meet if they only employed registered nurses.

Abel-Smith points out that nursing was virtually the only exclusively female profession at a time when the first wave of feminine emancipation began to rock the establishment at the end of the nineteenth century. Mrs Bedford Fenwick, one of the most active campaigners for nursing registration and a tireless worker for the establishment of nursing as a profession, was a well-known suffragette and an admirer of Mrs Pankhurst. For Bedford Fenwick, 'the nurse question was *the* woman question'; the nurse must be recognised as 'an individual of some importance in the state' (Abel-Smith 1975: 65). In her eyes, this could only be achieved by excluding the servant class of women, those who had traditionally undertaken nursing duties, from entry to the profession. Registration was seen not only as a means of conferring status on those who achieved it, but also as a means of controlling entry: admission had to be confined to the daughters of the higher social classes if nursing was to be recognised as a respectable profession separate from and free from the control of the medical establishment. Educational and financial barriers would ensure that only the better class of girl could become a nurse and 'undesirable' recruits (those from the lower social classes) would be kept out. At this time, nursing was still regarded by many in society as a disreputable occupation; one of the arguments used by Mrs Fenwick to drum up support for her campaign was that the richer classes needed to be protected from the criminal element in nursing. A registration scheme would ensure that this client group could be cared for in their own homes by nurses of good character.

Not all nursing leaders supported Mrs Fenwick and her organisation, the Royal British Nurses Association, in this quest; Nightingale herself was doubtful about the efficacy of the scheme, and considered 'good character' a more fitting attribute for prospective trainees irrespective of their social class, but by the end of the nineteenth century, her influence was diminishing. More forceful opposition to the Association's plans came from small provincial voluntary hospitals, where it was feared that the new regulations would make their own training schemes ineligible; they would therefore lose a valuable source of labour, as well as much of their local prestige. The Matrons of these institutions were worried that the creation of a nursing council to oversee training and registration would rob them of their local power bases. Others were against the exclusion of servants and lower-class girls from the nursing ranks, claiming that many of these young women made the best nurses because they were accustomed to servicing the needs of others.

These debates raged within the British nursing establishment between the years 1889 (when Bedford Fenwick established the British Nurses Association) and 1919, when the battle for registration was finally won. The feuds, now known as 'the thirty years war' in nursing history, left their marks on the profession inflecting the development of recruitment and staffing between the wars. Traditionally, nurse training was heavily concentrated in hospitals; how to provide enough nurses to staff these institutions was a continuing source of friction between the various nursing factions.

Before 1948 a three-tier system of administration consisting of the voluntary agencies, the local authority public health committees and the Poor Law or public assistance committees provided hospital services for the majority of the population (White 1985a). The first group had their roots in pre-Victorian and Victorian philanthropy, and were funded by upper-class benefactors and charitable donation. The second group developed through the Public Health movement and were charged with prevention of the spread of disease; many of these were known locally as fever hospitals. In the third group were institutions that cared for the chronic sick, aged and infirm, and the asylums which had their roots in nineteenth-century workhouse infirmaries. The status of these hospitals, and of their patients, and of the nurses who cared for them was intricately connected with their origins, as were the working conditions and salary arrangements between the three tiers.

The voluntary hospitals operated as autonomous organisations, independent from government policy and control, although they were increasingly reliant on government funding to remain solvent. In these hospitals, the Matron was recognised as head of all nursing services including the training school; she was autonomous, reporting directly to the governors. In the other types of hospital funding came primarily from local rates which made them more susceptible to political intervention. The Matrons of these institutions were responsible to a medical superintendent, overall head of the municipal hospital, who reported to a local health committee or medical officer of health. The nurses working in these hospitals tended to be non-resident and were sometimes married, unlike in the voluntary hospitals where residency tended to be enforced and marriage often entailed resignation (White 1985a). In the asylums, nursing was seen as a custodial activity; the majority of the staff were male and working-class. The lady reformers, because of their class origins and the nature of the work, largely ignored these hospitals (Carpenter 1980).

The Nurses Registration Act of 1919 introduced a mandatory syllabus of training and common examinations for all nurses. A general register of nurses was set up, with a supplementary register for male nurses, mental and mental deficiency nurses, sick children's nurses and an open section for any other speciality, e.g. fever nurses. The General Nursing Council (GNC) controlled only basic nursing training until 1943, when a further Nurses Act empowered the registration of nurse tutors. By 1948, in spite of the efforts of the GNC and the College of Nursing to enforce a policy where all nurses shared the same basic training, there was still a very wide range of qualifications available for specific spheres of work. Specialities such as ophthalmic and tuberculosis nursing continued to maintain their own training programmes, and the traditional split between the three types of hospital care and their differing status had not been healed.

Professional divisions in the 1930s

During the 1930s, divisions in the profession were reflected by the wide variety of trade union and professional associations which tried to organise nurses and campaign on their behalf. The Second World War, like the First, again brought a degree of homogeneity to the profession, but discontents over pay, conditions of service, working conditions and educational standards for trainees continued to fester. Amongst activist organisations in the 1930s, Dingwall identifies three main groupings: the hospital managements' position which had strong representation from the voluntary sector; the College of Nursing; and the trade unions, which tended to be heavily concentrated in local authority-run hospitals (Dingwall *et al.* 1988). Dingwall sees the Lancet Commission, launched in December 1930 to investigate nursing shortages, as representative of the hospital managements' viewpoint. The Commission consisted of representatives primarily from the voluntary sector and included only two hospital Matrons. The aim of the Commission was to offer 'recommendations for making the [nursing] service more attractive to women suitable for this necessary work'. Heavily biased towards the special circumstances of the voluntary sector, the report alleged that nursing was losing out to business, social work and teaching as a suitable form of employment for well-educated and therefore, at this time, inevitably, middle- and upper-class young women. Dingwall argues that it is unlikely that such women ever became nurses in anything like substantial numbers, and he points to a lack of statistical evidence for the claims made by the Lancet Commission. By 1939, the Athlone Committee was able to demonstrate that recruits were mainly culled from clerks, typists and shop assistants – the lower middle and respectable working classes (Dingwall *et al.* 1988: 99). This evidence is not dissimilar to the pattern of recruitment in late Victorian England found by Maggs (1983) and Simnett (1986) indicating that the principal pool of nursing labour was drawn from those who sought middle-class status and respectability. The Lancet report did serve to point out that petty rules and regulations, particularly in nurses' homes, tended to make the profession unattractive to young women living away from home. By the 1930s, the attitudes of many parents were a good deal more relaxed than those of their Victorian forebears; nonetheless, authoritarian practices both on the wards and in nurses' homes continued to dominate many trainee nurses' lives. These attitudes survived until the 1970s in spite of recommendations in numerous government reports that they should be abolished or amended.[2]

The College of Nursing saw itself as the representative voice of the leaders of the profession, and had worked hard to achieve this status. Founded in 1916 on the strength of the registration movement (although Mrs Bedford Fenwick was not a wholehearted supporter), the College was formally constituted along the lines of the Royal College of Physicians and

Surgeons in the hope of achieving comparable professional respectability for nursing. Its initial aims were to promote education and training, to introduce a uniform curriculum, to recognise approved training schools and to lobby Parliament in respect of nursing and health policies. Trade unionism of any sort or form was specifically banned from its articles of association (Abel-Smith 1975). Male nurses and mental nurses were excluded from membership, in much the same way that they were later to be excluded from the general nursing register. The College became a focus for the registration movement as its membership grew, and was finally in competition with the views of the Royal British Nurses Association led by Bedford Fenwick. The failure of these two groups to agree on the presentation of a joint Registration Bill eventually led to the then Minister of Health deciding to present a government bill in 1919. The passing of this Act gave the College dominant membership of the General Nursing Council; it was at this point that the College became indisputably the representative voice of the profession, a position it was to consolidate throughout the 1930s against a growing challenge from the trade union movement.

One of the ways that the College tried to recruit young women into the nursing profession in the 1930s was through writing for popular middle-class weekly magazines like *The Zodiac*. Agnes Pavey was a well-known commentator on nursing affairs and a nursing historian who supported the aims and objectives of the College.[3] In an undated article for *The Zodiac* lodged in the RCN archives, Pavey stresses the advantages of nursing in relation to other professions which had recently opened their doors to women. Asking why nursing is an unpopular profession today, she claims that it suffers from an 'over-emphasis on the vocational aspect that followed the work of Florence Nightingale'. In her brief account of the profession's unpopularity, she blames 'lurid press coverage' for persistently failing to differentiate between students and staff in matters of salary, perhaps a direct reference to media reportage of the 1937 campaign for higher salaries led by the unions. Through her dismissal of these campaigns, Pavey situates herself as a professionaliser, one of the group identified by Abel-Smith (1975) and Dingwall *et al.* (1988) whose values and attitudes were formed through association with the prestigious voluntary hospitals.

The photographs chosen to illustrate her article share the terms of reference in the text, emphasising a similarly high cultural, middle-class ethos. Centred on the opening page is a photograph of a nurse writing or sketching on a notepad, a skeleton hanging in front of her; the traditional relationship between artist and sitter is here reversed – the woman, usually the passive recipient of the (male) artist's objectification, controls the gaze.[4] Instead of the (male) doctor studying human remains for the pursuit of knowledge, the nurse occupies that position. On the second page of the article, two photographs are composed and lit similarly to an eighteenth-century Dutch still life painting; an image entitled 'Assisting the Surgeon' is composed and lit in a style that resembles Rembrandt's famous depiction of an anatomy lesson.[5] The classical references project a conception of occupational identity that exploits the divisions of labour in health care through a rubric of 'professionalism'. Two further images strengthen this impression, one of a senior nurse (wearing the cap and bow, a sign of her status) supervising junior nurses preparing food, and one of a nurse tending infants. Nursing, in Pavey's terms, is a 'separate but equal' sphere that converts feminine cultural capital (the often unpaid skills of food preparation and infant care) into social and economic capital.

In contrast, a trade union campaigning document from the mid-1930s combines an image of supplicancy with demands for better living conditions and wages for trainee nurses. The labour movement saw in the unregulated municipal hospital sector an opportunity to expand and develop its membership base; many general and white collar unions set out to recruit nurses during the 1930s (Hart 1994). The National Association of Local Government Officers (NALGO) was one of the unions that saw in the Lancet Commission's report an opportunity to recruit members by formulating 'a comprehensive recruitment and training scheme for women engaged in the Public Health Services'. Their *Women Public Health Workers' Charter* (1935) was addressed to nurses and was particularly concerned with nurse training and career development. The one-portal system of entry to the profession favoured by the College of Nursing and its supporters was a deterrent to young women from the respectable working class who wanted to become nurses. Many were denied a nursing career because of the gap in educational provision between the standard school leaving age and the commencement of training at 18. The report claimed that 'the young woman of today ... is physically and mentally several years ahead of the pre-war girl' and that 'the system must be made to conform to modern requirements if for no other reason than that comparatively few parents can afford to continue their girls' education up to 18 years of age' (*A Woman's Calling*, NALGO Women's Charter, 1935).

The image used by the union on the front of the brochure is interesting because it does not use the nursing uniform or any visual signifiers that might immediately call to mind the Nightingale ideal. It depicts a woman wearing ordinary everyday clothes; a small sketch of a classical building overprinted with a large cross (the emergency medical service symbol) occupies the lower right hand corner of the picture. The woman looks out over the reader's right shoulder, her arms outstretched and palms turned outwards, a pose suggesting supplicancy, service, vocation. Coupled with the large capital lettering across the top of the page and the dominance of the cross, the overall impression given by the cover is of a religious manifesto rather than a campaigning political document. Katherine Williams points out that the word 'calling', used in the title of the document, has a history in nursing that dates back to Nightingale's definition of nursing:

'they call it a profession, but I say that it is a calling' (Williams 1978). 'Calling' involves total submission and eradication of the self; the use of this term, combined with religious signifiers, aims to raise the political consciousness of the vocationalist element of the nursing workforce and convince them that they deserve a better deal. The manifesto combines a traditional image of female servitude with modern (feminist) demands for better pay and working conditions to win support for its campaign. The campaign replays the split in nursing that became apparent even in Nightingale's day – a split that led her to voice her disapproval of her rivals, and in particular of Bedford Fenwick and her feminist sympathies. Whereas Fenwick's efforts had been geared towards making nursing an exclusive profession for middle- and upper-class women in support of a liberal feminist agenda for equal access to the professions, NALGO's campaign uses the same terms of reference in an attempt to achieve equality of access for young women from lower-class backgrounds.

In 1937, a co-ordinating committee of the Trades Union Congress (TUC) combined a series of well-organised demonstrations with the issue of a Nurses Charter; extensive press coverage (Pavey's 'lurid publicity') prompted the Ministry of Health to establish the first comprehensive inquiry into nurses' pay and conditions.[6] War was again the motor that drove the government to intervene in nursing affairs by enacting the standardised payments scheme recommended in the Nurses Charter. The government passed legislation enabling staff to move quickly from one location to another as determined by need, unhindered by pay differentials. Rival factions within the nursing profession were unable to agree on either the pay scales or the implementation of a regularised scheme; the government imposed its solution in the form of the Rushcliffe Committee, which produced its first report in 1943. In spite of its opposition to government interference into pay and conditions the (by now) Royal College of Nursing (RCN) had a majority of seats on the staff side of the negotiations, and finally achieved their aim of widening the pay differentials between unqualified and qualified nurses (Dingwall *et al.* 1988: 104). Recruitment became the responsibility of the Ministry of Labour, who continued to organise national campaigns until 1957.

During the war years, there was general agreement within the coalition government that there should be some sort of comprehensive health service established that would cover all forms of curative and preventative treatment. The reforms became law in 1946, but much of the structure of health service provision was left largely intact; because of this the attitudes, working practices and culture of major institutions remained intact. The NHS Act established fourteen regional hospital boards and 388 hospital management committees; each committee was responsible for a group of hospitals organised according to geographical factors and medical function. Medical teaching hospitals were allowed to retain their autonomy and report directly to the Minister of Health. Large voluntary hospitals tended to remain relatively independent within hospital management committee groupings, or easily dominated the group in terms of administration, organisation, policy making and planning (White 1985a: 3). Some of the old 'Poor Law' institutions became residential homes, thus obviating the need for trained nursing staff and demoting those who worked in them to the status of attendants, or social service officers. In nursing terms, this meant that there was no radical shake-up of ideas and beliefs amongst the various factions, even though they were faced with what was potentially the most challenging period in their history. White (1985a) argues that nursing organisations were entirely omitted from the consultative process, implying that they were 'left out'. Dingwall claims that 'there is little evidence of pressure from nursing organisations for consultation on this, or indeed on any other aspect of early NHS legislation or policy', adding that there was 'considerable opposition [from the ministry] to appointing people in any sort of representative capacity' (Dingwall *et al.* 1988: 107).

Towards the end of the war, the National Advisory Council on Nurses and Midwives undertook to research and report on the training of nurses, commenting on the serious shortage of trainees and calling for substantial improvements in their treatment and training. Many of the Advisory Council's recommendations were adopted by the Wood Report, a government working party set up in 1946 to examine the recruitment and training of nurses. At this time there were over 11,000 vacancies for trained staff, 2,200 more than qualified each year from all parts of the register (White 1985a: 4). Accepting that there was a need to increase recruitment from secondary schools, the working party also recommended that girls leaving elementary education should be accepted for training to make up the shortfall. The report set the agenda for the way the Ministry of Health was to regard the position of nurses in the new NHS. A government circular in 1948, *Nursing and Domestic Staff in Hospitals: Notes for Guidance of HMCs* [Hospital Management Committees], treated nursing and domestic staff alike in respect of their workloads with few hints on what tasks should be undertaken by domestics rather than nurses; this report set the stage for the way nurses were treated by the ministry until the early 1960s (White 1985a). The implications of government intervention and control can be traced in relation to recruitment images used on brochures and leaflets in the 1950s.

Class divisions: job or profession?

Although many senior nurses were in favour of the NHS, some were not; the same sort of splits and divides that had caused divisions in the profession since 'the thirty years war' over registration were still operative. The teaching hospitals and the large voluntary hospitals (sometimes the same institution) regarded themselves as the professional elite of the medical world, recruiting their nursing staff from the independent and grammar school sector. These elite schools of nursing often had long waiting lists and tended to accept trainees on the basis of personal recommendation; many were the daughters of doctors and other professional people.[7] The large municipal hospitals drew recruits from their immediate geographical locality, supplementing their intake with recruits from overseas, particularly in the psychiatric sector. The shortage of trained staff continued to cause concern throughout the 1950s; Matrons travelled abroad in search of recruits, and incentives were given in the form of travel grants and bursaries to young women and men to come to Britain to train. Few incentives were offered to British-born men, however, other than to train for traditional male specialities; men in general nursing were few and far between, most having attained their qualifications during the war as part of the military medical corps. Active recruitment of men for general nursing began in the late 1960s, but the problems of recruitment and attrition continued unabated until high unemployment filled schools of nursing for the first time in 1975.

A number of research projects were initiated to study problems of recruitment and attrition, most of which adopted a functionalist approach. Often undertaken by university sociology and psychology departments, the aim of this research was to locate the 'ideal type' of young woman who was suitable for nursing and target her for recruitment.[8] The research methods focused on the personality traits of individuals who 'failed' to adapt to nursing; this had particular implications for black nurses, discussed below in greater detail. The nursing schools, their institutional cultures, training and employment practices were not considered part of an equation for successful staff retention.[9] Intellect was not the most important quality in a prospective nurse, reflecting the values of the dominant group in nursing at this time, the 'generalists', and their influence on the principal official body, the GNC.

The 'generalists' attitudes and values were similar to those of Nightingale; they favoured targeting for training 'the servant class', respectable working-class girls who had no difficulty serving others. From the 'professionals' point of view this approach lowered educational standards; they maintained higher entry standards to the elite schools of nursing in an attempt to retain their control of the profession. These internal disputes created a narrowness of vision amongst nursing leaders which was reinforced by the research commissioned by the Department of Health. The government, as numerous reports showed, considered nursing a semi-skilled job. There was no real incentive for them to be seriously concerned about staffing the hospitals with trained nurses because the bill for nurses' wages was the highest cost the NHS had to bear. A constant stream of young women in training was the cheapest way to staff the wards. This attitude probably accounts for the total lack of research interest in actual working conditions, such as long hours, split shifts and night duty, and the failure to initiate change.

In the United States, less functionally orientated research began to high-light different attitudes to work amongst nurses. Habenstein and Christ (1955) identified three main types of nurse with very different conceptual frameworks of their role. The first, the professionaliser, was preoccupied with medico-scientific and nursing knowledge and tended to be more inter-ested in curing diseases than caring for the patient. The second, the traditionaliser, matches the stereotype of much popular fiction, supporting a vocational ideology of 'tender loving care'; notions of selfless devotion to patients and a deferential 'handmaiden' attitude to medical practitioners predominate in this group. The third type, the utiliser nurse, 'is the proto-type of the nurse as a piece rate worker, a low-level non-professional organisational employee who simply does her job' (Matz (1969) in Mercer 1979: 136). Within the British context, these ideas translate into three dominant ideologies: nursing as a profession, nursing as a vocation, and nursing as a custodial activity (K. Williams 1978). Vocational ideology trans-forms the relationship between patient and caretaker from one based in hierarchical divisions of class authority to one based on gender difference through the metaphor of the idealised middle-class family, where sexual difference can be controlled because the nurse is a literal or metaphorical mother (Poovey 1989: 184–5). The patient's dignity is preserved by the knowledge that his child-like state of dependency is tended by somebody who considers it a privilege rather than a duty to serve him. Basic nursing care (feeding, washing and attending to bodily functions) in the absence of antibiotics and antisepsis could and sometimes did save the lives of those who might otherwise have died. As Williams points out, the training curriculum which established certain bedside nursing tasks as essential for the well-being of the patient (bed baths, feeding and toileting) also transformed the status of the sick. No part of a sick person's body was ever unnecessarily exposed during these processes by a nurse of worth and sensitivity. Although the helpless sick adult 'may have lost *his* [*sic*] independence, *his* worth as a person is increased by the nurse's dedication to tasks performed in willing service to helplessness' (Williams 1978: 40, my emphasis).

Vocational ideology masks the gender hierarchy built into the doctor/ nurse relationship, and the powerlessness of the patient. Professional ideology, on the other hand, demands that the nurse be highly skilled, rather than selfless and dedicated to her work. Notions of humanitarian service and eradication of the self stand in stark opposition to ideas of self-worth, status and personal autonomy. The professional nurse is more concerned with curing than caring; this emphasis tends to objectify the patient and his illness into a mass of clinical terms and judgements (Dingwall *et al.* 1988). The adult condition of helplessness experienced by the patient is treated by the nurse as a clinical state; how the patient feels is less important than knowing the correct clinical labels, monitoring increasingly complex technology, and carrying out intricate clinical procedures and observations. Formerly skilled tasks, such as the monitoring of bodily temperature by thermometer and bedside care, are relegated to those who are less skilled, and therefore cheaper to employ. Williams argues that an ideology of vocation 'becomes dysfunctional or obsolete where skilled tasks require judgement rather than obedience, and since the acquisition of skills has to be paid for, the tasks to which they relate cannot then be regarded by society, doctors or nurses as menial . . . seen as skilled they require an assertion of self in creative and innovative action' (Williams 1978: 41). A professional concern and interest with the clinical side of curing tends to be biased in favour of nursing the 'crisis' and then rescinding care of the patient to those who are less skilled. If the person continues to remain in a state of helplessness (i.e. is deemed incurable), he or she is likely to be transported to an institution where long-term care will be provided by groups other than the 'professional' nurse. The helpless sick adult, whose consciousness of her/his condition will vary in relation to the degree of impairment experienced, is likely to receive custodial care which, according to Williams, 'evaluates helplessness in adults as a regression to infant behaviours' (1978: 43). Although Williams does not draw the parallel, the ideology of this group may well have its roots in the disenfranchisement from nursing culture they experienced as successive waves of professional activity have sought to exclude handywomen, nursing auxiliaries and other carers from nursing's professional institutions.[10]

Williams' approach to the divisions in nursing focuses on the helpless individual as the focal point of the definitions. In contrast, White takes an institutional approach, arguing that the ideologies of nursing in place by the mid-1970s were as dependent upon their institutional base within the hospital system as they were a century earlier (White 1985b). Her analysis of political regulators in British nursing provides an added dimension to the changes brought about by nationalisation (White 1985b). She identifies three main interest groups in nursing: the managers, the specialists (or professionalists) and the generalists. The generalists are those who maintain that nursing is a practical occupation, that academic and intellectual qualifications are not necessary, that there is no need of a theoretical base and that first-level training to registration standard is all that is needed by way of preparation. The term describes an occupational ideology where the members are class-conscious, accepting of a hierarchy, and, similarly to 'utilisers', used to performing unskilled or semi-skilled tasks under the supervision of a specialist or manager. This group are more likely to join trade unions for solidarity and negotiating power, and insist on practical experience as a criterion for promotion. The specialists or professionals seek to maintain control over their work, working without the supervision of other nurses; they take additional qualifications and try to achieve expert status within their chosen speciality. Although this conception of nursing work challenges the hierarchical structure of nursing, they favour the administration of nursing via nurse managers whom they also expect to be specialists within their chosen field. Specialists, as White points out, respect and acknowledge specialists in other fields. The nurse managers are the planners and policy makers, and work within a multi-disciplinary bureaucratic framework where the culture of management predominates. To be effective, they must have power, and power is bought through the application of management rather than nursing skills. This group has a history of trying to control nursing by attention to manpower (*sic*) needs, suppressing the development of specialists and professional education in the interests of economy. White claims that this group feels challenged by the authority of the professionals and is more at ease with the generalists who are unlikely to question the hierarchical status quo. The power and authority at one time invested in the image of the voluntary hospital Matron are split here into two separate nursing identities. One has the power to hire and fire nursing staff, but no authority in the specialist areas of nursing knowledge; the other is an 'authority' in her chosen area of expertise, but her power is confined to developing her own speciality and participating in nurse education (White 1985b).

These three groups, with their various strategies for seeking status and different definitions of what that status actually entails, form the three main interest groups in nursing in post-war England. In 1950, twenty-six out of the thirty-six members of the General Nursing Council took their seats for the first time. Half of these were newly elected representatives, and half were newly appointed. White identifies a profound change in the composition of this group, which was not appreciated at the time. Senior nurses on the earlier GNC had trained before educational entry requirements were relaxed to meet war-time need, and tended to promote professionalisation through recruiting candidates from secondary schools and raising the standards of nurse training. In 1944/45 they had attempted to re-introduce a minimum entry qualification, relaxed during war-time to meet staffing needs. Many who sat on the 1950 GNC entered nursing through the open recruitment policy introduced in 1938; in their eyes, the need for labour for the newly nationalised health service was of greater importance than raising educational standards.

It was not until 1959 that the Ministry of Health agreed to a resumption of educational entry requirements, by which time the values of many of the Matrons had undertaken a subtle shift, from one of service to the patient to one of service to the NHS. This new ethic, termed by White 'the common good', became the basis for all future decision making. One of the effects of this change was to lower the entry standard for nursing from its pre-war requisite of five subjects passed in consolidated examination, to a two 'O' level minimum which could be taken serially. In White's opinion, the GNC changed from being an instrument of education to being an instrument of recruitment, becoming an agent of the government and employing authorities (White 1985b: 26).[11] White is highly critical of the role played by the major representative bodies of nursing – the GNC, the staff side of the Whitley pay negotiating council, the Standing Nurses Advisory Committee and the council of the RCN. She claims that the Matrons, selected by the Ministry of Health and the employing institutions, were chosen because they followed the line of acting in the 'common good'. Revealing her professional sympathies, White exclaims 'I recall no occasion when the argument of "for the good of the profession" prevailed' (White 1985b: 30). The generalists, along with managers, are seen as luddite-like in their endorsement of the common good, the by-product of which was a de-skilling of the nursing workforce and the employment of a generalist level of labour. Recruitment images from the 1950s are analysed below with White's account very much in mind. What are the differences between recruitment images for state registration and state enrolment? And what effect did the labour shortage have on the way young women were encouraged to regard nursing work?

Recruitment images in the 1950s

The nurse depicted on the cover of the Ministry of Labour's 1950 recruitment brochure *Your Chance* is a far cry from her traditional Nightingale counterpart; she is young and attractive with fashionably arched brows and short wavy hair. Her address to the reader is very direct; she looks out with an open, smiling mouth, the darkness of which is suggestive of lipstick. The short-sleeved uniform with white collar and apron is drawn with shadowing indicative of soft fabric folds; her hat sits neatly on top of her head, leaving much of her hair exposed. Drawn from the side to accentuate her feminine curves, she is caught in motion, her face turned to glance at the reader as she 'flies by' with her tray. The image bears a startling resemblance to dust cover pictures of Cherry Ames, the popular American nurse featured in career novels. Behind her, there is a clipboard pinned to the wall and some flowers sketched in – the one indicative of her observational and recording role, the other of her femininity. There has always been an element of surprise in the response at conferences and seminars that this image is a representation of a nurse; many people read the woman as a waitress and presume she is carrying a tray of food.

The idea of 'waiting on' someone, although it dominates the cover, tends to be refuted in the second image which depicts the hospital staff – surgeons, radiographers, domestic staff, dieticians, bacteriologists, almoners, masseuses – in a series of circular photographs with two nurses at the

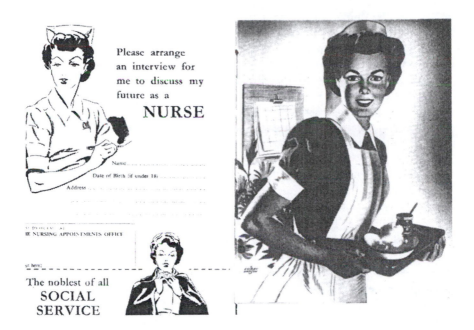

Figure 3.1 Recruitment leaflet *Your Chance*, 1950s (Ministry of Labour/Central Office of Information)

centre. In this atomic vision of the health care team, nurses are the nucleus on whom all else depends. Other images depict nurses administering medicines and teaching students; rows of trainee nurses sit in identical positions writing notes. Under the heading 'A distinguished career' the reader is informed that nursing 'offers scope for advancement rarely equalled in an ordinary job, as distinct from a professional post', and told about senior posts 'of great responsibility in the service of the nation'. The text is at pains to stress improved conditions of service and describes how time will be spent during training. At the bottom is a list of questions and answers: What happens if I fall ill, fail the exams, get married before or after qualification? The concluding paragraph assures the reader that 'the experience you have gained as a nurse will be of life long value' and, if you do decide to carry on nursing after you are married, 'there are many openings available to you which you can combine with your household responsibilities'. In the final photograph, a large group of nurses (perhaps at a graduation ceremony or similar event because they are not wearing aprons) present an image of drilled uniformity. Facing this photograph is a sketch of a nurse holding a child wrapped in a blanket with a bandaged head; in the background a child is sitting up in bed. Below it are described two other ways to become a nurse through state enrolment.

A closer examination of the signifying systems of this brochure reveals some interesting dichotomies. The back page is similar in style to the front, although the nurses pictured are sketched rather than drawn in detail. The word 'nurse', printed in large capital letters, is the boldest of the images on the page, and matches the scripting style of the brochure's final statement, 'The noblest of all social service for a woman'. Like the word 'nurse', 'social service' is presented in capitals, one word below the other, reiterating the idea of service presented on the cover. The photographs present an interesting formal contrast to the informality of the sketches. In the drawings, which begin and end the booklet, the nursing figures look soft, small featured and feminine. The woman on the cover looks out cheekily and invitingly; confident and assured, her gaze meets ours. In the sketch on the last inside page the nurse holding the child has lowered lids, her dropped gaze posing a submissive, maternal look as she protectively holds the child, one hand adjusting the blanket. On the back cover, there is a return to the confident glance of the cover girl, only her gaze is directed slightly away from the reader. She is writing in fountain pen on a clipboard, looking professional, detached and slightly aloof. In contrast the photographs, unlike those found in popular middle-class news magazines of the time such as *Picture Post*,[12] are formally composed; uniformity of stance and posture suggests that these shots are arranged. Everything is too rigid, too tidy with no hint of spontaneity. All the photographs share this rigid formal style, a referential ethos that also pervades the recruitment films commissioned by the Central Office of Information.

The formal style of these pictures indicates that deliberate choices were made about the kind of representations that were desirable, but the overall message of the brochure is in some ways a contradictory one. The sketched images depict a fun-loving figure that disappears into a rather cool, more sophisticated creature by the final pages. A journey from innocence to experience is charted through images of training and discipline, suggesting perhaps that becoming a nurse will transform you from an ordinary 'girl next door' into a middle-class professional. Becoming a nurse entails a change in social status, and with that status comes a confident detachment. The government are attempting to represent nursing through a combination of official (formal) discourse and popular images in an attempt to broaden their address, but the awkward juxtaposing of these two formations of nursing identity eventually resulted in the production of separate materials for the two different tiers of training.

In the post-war period, the Ministry of Labour continued to produce information on careers for dissemination to schools, labour exchanges and career offices. *Nursing and Midwifery Services* (women) was No. 33 in their 'Careers for Men and Women' series. The booklet has 38 pages, most of which are text; photographs, many of them identical to the ones used in *Your Chance*, pepper the pages which suggests that most of the material for the smaller leaflet was drawn from this one. Half of this publication deals with training, the rest of it with career prospects for qualified nurses and midwives in Britain and abroad as a member of the armed forces.

Leaflets produced by the Nursing Recruitment Service set a different tone from the government publications, partly because they are text-based and have no photographs, although the basic information is the same. Organised by the nursing profession (rather than the government) through the King Edward's Hospital Fund for London, the service provided an alternative source of information on training at the London teaching hospitals.[13] Future leaders of the profession were traditionally trained in these institutions; King's Fund brochures direct their address to academic young women attending grammar schools who might consider nursing as a career rather than just a job. The leaflet produced in the early 1950s emphasises the 'social value' and 'absorbing interest' of nursing; assistant nurse training is recommended for those 'who would find state examination too difficult', rather than as a separate field dedicated to nursing the chronic sick and elderly. A question about educational standards emphasises the scope in the profession for those of 'marked ability and high educational standard', while pointing out that low educational attainment does not prevent a girl from becoming a nurse. The overall tone of the leaflet is geared towards attracting well-educated grammar school girls irrespective of high academic attainment, projecting a very different image from the official publications. These are most marked in relation to attitudes to SEN training, the portal of entry created by the GNC in 1943 to recognise the grade of assistant nurse. In the Ministry of Labour brochure, training for this grade is described beneath a picture of a nurse holding a child, emphasising the 'maternal' nature of this kind of work. Glamour and maternal values work hand in hand on the brochure to indicate the feminine nature of the work, but in reality, for all its rewards, the work was physically demanding and often 'dirty'. Whilst the child can be read as a metaphor for the helpless patient, for the girl who is thinking of becoming an assistant nurse, caring for children is probably a more attractive proposition than caring for helpless elderly adults, as Jeffery's (1950) research indicated. At no point in any of the literature is there any indication just how separate the two tiers of nursing are; not only was training for each grade carried out in different types of hospitals, but the working conditions of the two groups were barely comparable. It is this element of nursing work that the professionalisers have always sought to distance themselves from, seeking, as White (1985b) has pointed out, expertise in the area of acute care where curing has a higher value than caring, and personal autonomy is developed through specialisation.

Gender divisions: men enter the picture

It was not only divisions between different classes of nurse that fractured professional unity; with the admission of men to the general registration roll in 1949, another powerful interest group quickly developed. Men are virtually absent from popular and professional images of the period, but their impact at all levels of the profession was significant. The gendered divisions in health care situate nursing as women's work, but there have always been male nurses – in psychiatric nursing, in the prison services and in the armed forces. Professionalisation in nursing developed in general nursing, an area dominated by women, and from which men were effectively excluded until the admission of men to the register in 1949. Men were not permitted to join the Royal College of Nursing until 1960; they become visible in the recruitment literature from the mid-1960s, but they were not actively recruited in mass campaigns until the end of the decade. Was this increasing visibility of men due to a small but vocal male faction who had made their way into the higher echelons of the profession by this time? As White (1985a) notes, many men entered general nursing during the Second World War via the armed services. At the end of the war, some of them switched to civilian nursing, increasing the percentage of men in hospital nursing overall, especially in psychiatric care, but in addition the numbers of men in general nursing grew quite significantly. Mrs H was Principal Nursing Officer (Education) at the United Liverpool Hospitals throughout the 1960s. In an interview discussing nurse recruitment, she pointed out that she had 'never worked with a male colleague in my training or subsequently until I went to do the Sister Tutor's course [note Sister – they were still called Sister Tutors in those days] between 1955 and 57. There were several men on the course and they had come from the psychiatric field and the general field – the ones in the general field had all been in the forces' (January 1992). While on this course, she met Mr R, later in charge of recruitment for the Broadgreen group of hospitals in Liverpool. Mr R was an army-trained general nurse who held senior nursing rank in the Royal Army Medical Corps. After the war, he had to find a hospital where men were accepted for general nurse training – at this time, there were about twelve in Britain and only a handful of hospitals employed qualified male nurses. The salaries for ex-service personnel were paid by a post-war government resettlement scheme; hospitals with severe staffing problems took advantage of the scheme and accepted male entrants, as well as trawling abroad for overseas applicants (Mr R, personal communication, 1992).

Many men entered general nursing through the former municipal hospitals where there was a greater tendency towards unionisation amongst the rank and file and a managerialist ethos to the provision of nursing care. By 1950 there were 25,600 male nurses in a total nursing population of 152,000 –

just over 16 per cent; five men were now sitting on the GNC out of a total of thirty-six representatives. Throughout the 1950s and 1960s male nurses consistently achieved senior posts in general nursing in spite of the fact that there were fewer of them undertaking training. The reasons for this are generally attributed to the different career aspirations of men and women in nursing. In their analysis of a group of male student nurses in 1968, Brown and Stones identified a difference in attitudes to nursing between male entrants and female entrants. Although educational background was a factor in male attitudes to nursing, it was a much less significant factor than amongst female recruits and school leavers. The male entrants, irrespective of educational background (although their education level was generally lower than that of female entrants), tended to see nursing as a career rather than a job or a vocation. They were more career-minded, seeing a path of progression before them even before they had completed the basic training. Brown and Stones point out that 'it could be that men needed the career image to rationalise and legitimise (to themselves and their peers) their decision to enter a field that, as they themselves said, was not thought of as a man's job and was moreover poorly paid'. Significantly, men who did not have a career vision tended to leave before completing their training, having decided that nursing was not for them (Brown and Stones 1973: 80).

Male entrants do seem to have been more career-orientated than their female counterparts from the outset, no doubt because of their social conditioning which placed an emphasis on the role of the male as economic provider. There was still an expectation amongst young women that nursing was a 'fill-in' between school and marriage – an attitude reflected in the recruitment literature. For many young women, this was undoubtedly the case; numbers of qualified female nurses dropped dramatically after the age of 25, the age at which promotion and progression started to be considered. Since men were (and still are) highly likely to stay in the profession once they have trained, they quickly became over-represented in middle management levels in relation to their numbers overall. Brown and Stones argued at this time that 'Men offer an important alternative to the traditional spinster in all fields of nursing ... marriage is more likely to bind men to a career than to wean them from it ... once trained [men] can be counted as permanent additions to the hospital nursing staff' (1973: 25). Male recruitment was actively revived in 1968, in part due to the recession; during the Depression of the 1930s, men had similarly sought nursing posts due to the shortage of other kinds of work (Brown and Stones 1973: 109). In casual conversation with male nurses on the wards in the 1980s, many of them claimed to have entered nursing due to a lack of other job opportunities in their immediate geographical area. Their choice of nursing as a career reflects work patterns in other areas of the economy – when jobs are in short supply, men take over the low status work traditionally done by women.

In spite of arguments for targeting males, the favoured recruitment group in English hospitals during the 1960s continued to be young unmarried women with middle-class backgrounds, a grammar school education and English parentage (Jones (1967) in Brown and Stones 1973). By 1965, the Nursing Recruitment Service had updated their recruitment literature very moderately. Perhaps they still felt that the reasons for maintaining a separate recruitment service to that run by the Ministry of Health were as pertinent as they were in the 1950s. The Service was one way of maintaining a separate image of professional identity at a time when the former voluntary hospitals, traditionally trainers of the leaders of the nursing profession, felt themselves to be under threat from the government's image of nursing. The recruitment leaflets produced by the Ministry of Health were not, as Mrs H pointed out during interview, an image of nursing approved of or used for recruiting people to traditional centres of excellence. The Nursing Recruitment Service continued to provide publications for these institutions, presenting nursing as a distinctly professional career for young middle-class women. By the 1960s there were some significant differences between their own earlier publications and the updated version, the most obvious of which is the addition of a picture on the front cover of the small brochure *Nursing Today*. It features a nurse sitting at a desk writing, her face and hands illuminated by a pool of light from an unseen desk lamp or similar light source. The framework of reference is quite unmistakable: here is the Lady of the Lamp, sitting with a concentrated air of autonomous authority, writing. The image continues to embody a particular set of ideas and values. The discourse inscribed on the image of this woman, with its unmistakable reference to the Nightingale ideal, emphasises education and scholarship, drawing on professional nursing's growing promotion of Nightingale as an administrator and a leader. This model of the professional nurse wears the trappings of vocational nursing, the white starched apron and the small lace hat of the Victorian maid, but for those experienced enough to decipher the hierarchical symbolism, she is at the very least a Sister, epitomising an ideal of female authority based on the notion of service – a 1960s version of the traditional 'angel'.

Inside its cover, the brochure is laid out similarly to its predecessor, using a question and answer format. Instead of the former emphasis on social service with its associated implication of nursing as women's work encapsulated in the phrase 'A girl who enters the nursing profession undertakes work of great social value', there is a more individuated ungendered opening address: 'People who become nurses can be assured that their work will be of real value to the community and a source of happiness and satisfaction to themselves.' The 'social' has been replaced by the concept of 'community', a word that has never had an unfavourable connotation although who or what that community is or might be is left for the reader to deduce. No longer do nursing and medicine contribute to 'the health services of

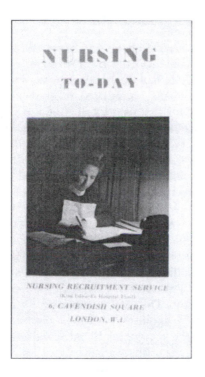

Figure 3.2 Recruitment leaflet *Nursing Today*, 1960s (Nursing Recruitment Service, King Edward's Hospital Fund)

the nation', but to the 'well-being of all'. The nationalist ethos of post-war Britain gives way to the rhetoric of consensus politics in the phrase 'mutual well-being', an indication of a changing conception of the role of the professional nurse. The new wording emphasises the separate but equal contribution of doctors and nurses to well-being with the implication that nurses are actively involved in the process of health care. Elizabeth Wilson, in her analysis of the position of women in post-war Britain, notes that the literature on marriage changes to a rhetoric of partnership and co-operation with an increased emphasis on togetherness, an updated middle-class ideal of separate spheres replacing the pre-war notion of women servicing the needs of their husbands (Wilson 1980). Given a model of health care with its roots in rigid gendered divisions of labour, it is unsurprising to find the rhetoric of professional nursing using the same metaphoric language as that of the literature on marriage. The small changes in the brochure can be seen as part of a more widespread cultural change in the discourse on women's role, rather than an active pursuit of change by the nursing profession. The overall message of this brochure echoes that of its predecessor; to do interesting nursing work, you have to be both educated and qualified (i.e. state registered).

Nowhere in the recruitment literature are the changes in nurse education mapped so clearly as when these two documents from the 1950s and 1960s are set side by side. Whereas previously it had been possible to train in numerous branches of nursing, now students are advised to start with a general qualification, since it is necessary for the majority of all senior posts. General nursing's progress towards hegemony in the education sector is by this stage completed. Experimental combined courses are mentioned, which result in joint qualifications in two fields after four years. Attention is also drawn to the new courses which combine general nursing and mid-wifery with public health and district nursing. Degree courses in Manchester and Edinburgh are available (but not in London, due to friction between the Royal College of Nursing and the University of London over course content). All the integrated and experimental courses demand university entrance standards. Some shortened courses are available for graduates and others with comparable educational qualifications.

Other material produced at this time by the Nursing Recruitment Service emphasises the modern ward environment. The architecture and furniture of hospital wards is often neglected as a significant factor in recruitment literature, the emphasis falling on modern conditions in nurses' homes in an attempt to compensate for their pre-war authoritarian image. As Karen Kingsley suggests, however, 'the built form reflects the social and cultural position of nursing' (Kingsley 1988: 63). In the brochure *Your Life in Nursing* the ward depicted has an intimate feel in comparison to the long 'Nightingale' wards common in Victorian hospitals. Bright curtains and flowers are a welcome visual distraction in the rather sparse environment, which shows four or five patients lying in their beds with two nurses and a white-coated figure attending them. A large picture of a young nurse occupies the left hand foreground. She gazes directly out from the page, appearing neither coquettish, nor coy, but serious and rather businesslike, with a hint of humour in the slightly up-turned corners of her mouth. Her uniform is a modern variant of the traditional format: white collar, apron and cuffs on a short-sleeved pinstripe button-through dress. Her hat sits neatly and unobtrusively on the back of her head. This rather ordinary young woman has perhaps been chosen as a suitable image for the brochure because of her serene quality. Placed as she is on the page, overlapping the main picture of the ward, she seems to belong to her environment in a quietly authoritative manner. Nursing seems less dominated in this image by the traditions of the past and is more integrally constituted as part of modern hospital life.

By the mid-1960s, the Ministry of Health and the Ministry of Labour were jointly producing recruitment materials. Leaflet NL 013 *You Want to Be a Nurse? Your Questions Answered* is in the tradition of its post-war predecessors, using cartoon sketches to create broad, lightweight appeal. The leaflet stands out because it is pale blue, which emphasises the comic nurse figures. The basic format is of a list of twenty questions with small ink-drawn cartoon sketches in the margins. The sketches parody patients, doctors and primarily nurses in a variety of 'typical' situations – taking a temperature, tending a mother and baby, attending lectures, relaxing in the nurses' home, and finally standing alone with a halo! The lighthearted, fun approach is similar to the cartoon style used to create the title sequence for the popular British *Doctor* films; the implication is that nursing is no longer stuck in the authoritarian ways of the past, it is a lively job where there is time to stand around and joke with your (male medical) colleagues. By this time, nursing was having to compete with other para-medical specialities such as physiotherapy and radiography for their share of the female labour market and had to take a more active, campaigning approach to recruitment. It seems likely that this brochure was used to appeal to those who may not necessarily consider working as a nurse.

During the same period, a brochure was circulating that clearly had more serious appeal. Again, it has a drawn cover, but this time the background paper is pink, and the style of line drawing resembles the kind of image that young women were accustomed to seeing in popular girls' magazines like *Bunty* and *Judy*. These magazines often had heroines who were highly active and successful, stressing individual achievement in fields like horse riding, skating, ballet and acting. Addressing the lower middle-class pre-teenage readership of *Bunty* and *Judy*, girls who are likely to be doing well at school as a result of the new meritocracy in education, the leaflet stresses that a first-class training is available not only in London and the large cities but at over 400 regional hospitals; 'there is certain to be one within fairly easy reach of your home'. Attempts were being made to spread the notion of excellence attached to the London teaching hospitals and their nursing schools throughout the regional hospital system as re-organisation of the health service sought to erode traditional centres of medical power in the interests of a more equitable distribution of services. Standing amidst a group of friends carrying books is a 'Sue Barton' look-alike, neat, professional and feminine but with no hint of sexual appeal. She is accompanied by a man, clearly signified as a nurse by his white buttoned tunic; in the background is a Palladian building. This re-formation of the cover of the 1950s 'Careers for Men and Women' brochure uses similar classical signifiers to suggest knowledge and professionalism. Like its predecessor, it is illustrated throughout with carefully posed photographs that show the various faces of nursing. Although there is a new emphasis on technical procedures, the overall impression is one of traditional values: concentrated faces lit by a desk lamp on night duty, mothering a small child, protectively watched over by a doctor/teacher, assisting the doctor in theatre. In the nurses' home, women (again, the nurses depicted are all female

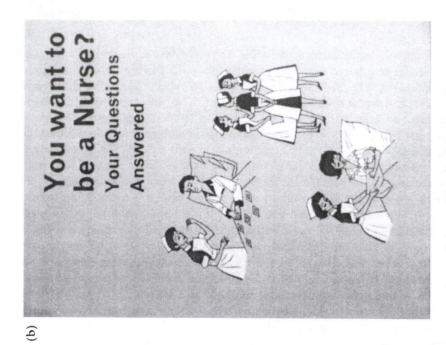

(b)

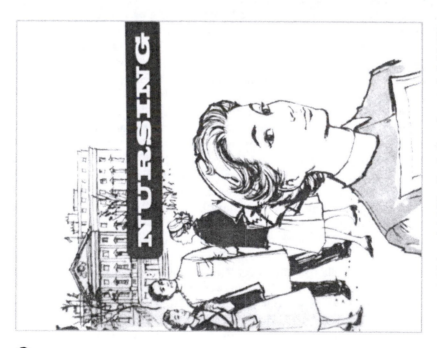

(a)

Figures 3.3(a) and 3.3(b) 'Classical' and 'popular' 1960s recruitment leaflets (Ministry of Labour/Ministry of Health/Central Office of Information)

apart from the figure on the cover) sit and play records and dance; the shortage of male partners is noticeable.

Two rather glossy brochures were produced at this time that adopted fashionable modes of presentation from popular magazines and advertising, signalling a new consciousness in government publications of the importance of visual images. These brochures foreground the use of photography far more consciously than their predecessors, using documentary and photojournalism techniques. This style of photography, long favoured by quality news publications, aims to capture 'life as it is', through live shooting. The overall effect is to inject a sense of urgency and dynamism previously absent from depictions of nursing work. Whereas previously pictures had served the purpose of illustrating particular situations and tasks, now the emphasis is on using the pictures to tell the story.

The full colour cover of the state registration brochure, labelled simply *SRN* in bright red lettering, shows a young woman in full uniform against the blurred, obviously moving, image of an ambulance behind her. This sense of urgency continues in the black and white photo-narrative that illustrates the process of training from the first interview with Matron to the final images of 'high-tech' medical care. Inside, a full page photo depicts the nurse looking at a white-coated male figure against the background of the ward, with a patient clearly visible. Against expectations, the man in the white coat is not a doctor but a charge nurse, her immediate superior and in charge of the ward team. This is the only depiction of a male nurse in the brochure; the same image was used in a cropped version on the front cover of *How to Become a Nurse: A Brief Guide for Men and Women*, leaflet HSC 102. The presence of men in general nursing is acknowledged as is, later in the brochure, the presence of a black nurse in training – the first time such images appear in the recruitment literature.

In this brochure, photographs dominate the written word, creating a photo story similar in style to those in contemporary girls' comics such as *Diana*.[14] The story of Patricia Dyer's training is mapped in captioned photos which emphasise varied work with patients, much of it looking fairly technical. The body of the patient is positioned centrally as the core of nursing work, which is presented as a series of tasks performed on the body; on many of the pictures, the patient's face cannot be seen. The effect of this dismemberment is to depersonalise the work, concealing the potential distastefulness of contact with bodily emissions. Objectification works hand in hand with melodramatic lighting to create an atmosphere similar to that of the popular television medical documentary series, *Your Life in Their Hands* (BBC 1 1958–64). In this series, the patient was scarcely seen, merely presented as a slab of flesh under the gown (Karpf 1988a: 55). This was the period when television concentrated on the dramatic, life-saving aspects of medicine – values that are exploited here by nursing recruiters. The overall tone of this brochure is completely

(a)

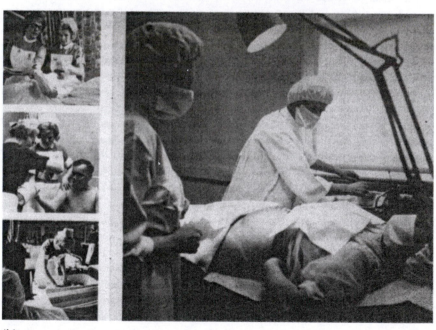

(b)

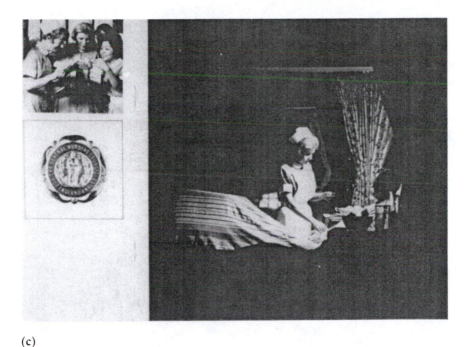

(c)

Figures 3.4(a), 3.4(b) and 3.4(c) SRN brochure, 1960s (Ministry of Labour/Ministry of Health/Central Office of Information)

different from that of its forerunners because of its visual qualities; the emphasis is on the role of the nurse in saving and preserving life, making nursing 'surely the most rewarding job in the world'. Information about training follows the narrative of the photographs, explaining the different stages leading to state registration. There are few headings, so the one labelled 'training after marriage' stands out. For the first time it is theoretically possible to marry during training and live out, although in practice this was still discouraged in many training schools.

A separate brochure was produced to recruit trainees for the roll, *Proud Badge of Service: A Close Look at the Rewarding Job of an Enrolled Nurse*. The colour photography cover depicts an attractive 'Audrey Hepburn' look-alike model pinning a badge to her uniform. A very different formation of nursing identity is apparent in this brochure; although a similar photo-narrative technique is used to illustrate the training process, it lacks the excitement of the SRN publication. The photographs are more evenly lit, depicting tasks performed in a modern hospital setting. Sketches undermine the seriousness of the brochure, creating an impressionistic lighthearted approach to the subject and removing much of the melodramatic intensity

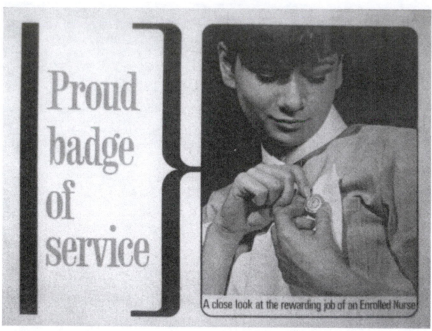

Proud badge of service

A close look at the rewarding job of an Enrolled Nurse

(a)

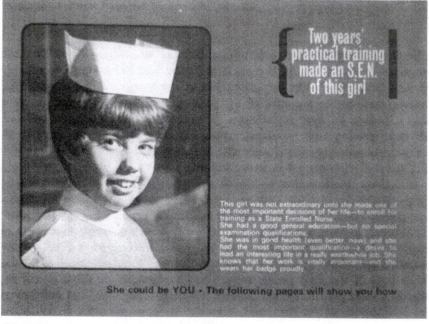

Two years' practical training made an S.E.N. of this girl

This girl was not extraordinary until she made one of the most important decisions of her life—to enroll for training as a State Enrolled Nurse.
She had a good general education—but no special examination qualifications.
She was in good health (even better now) and she had the most important qualification—a desire to lead an interesting life in a really worthwhile job. She knows that her work is vitally important—and she wears her badge proudly.

She could be YOU · The following pages will show you how

(b)

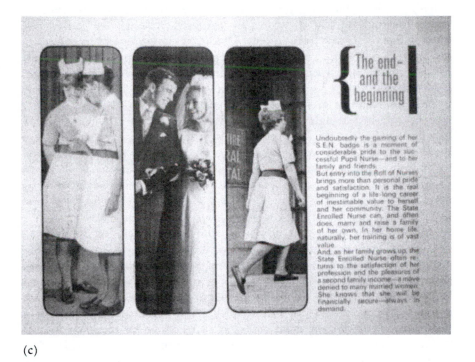

The end – and the beginning

Undoubtedly the gaining of her S.E.N. badge is a moment of considerable pride to the successful Pupil Nurse—and to her family and friends. But entry into the Roll of Nurses brings more than personal pride and satisfaction. It is the real beginning of a life-long career of inestimable value to herself and her community. The State Enrolled Nurse can, and often does, marry and raise a family of her own. In her home life, naturally, her training is of vast value. And, as her family grows up, the State Enrolled Nurse often returns to the satisfaction of her profession and the pleasures of a second family income—a move denied to many married women. She knows that she will be financially secure—always in demand.

(c)

Figures 3.5(a), 3.5(b) and 3.5(c) Proud Badge of Service, SEN brochure, 1960s (Ministry of Labour/Ministry of Health/Central Office of Information)

achieved by the documentary photo-narrative. The first page contains the rather surprising words, 'She may or may not be a natural beauty. Either way, she's attractive to everyone because she's confident and poised', with a photograph of the back view of a nurse walking away from the camera. This is followed by the caption, 'Two years practical training made an SEN of this girl' adjacent to a close-up of a rather cheeky looking young woman with buck teeth. The sub-text is clear: physical attractiveness is not a precondition for nursing! The text emphasises the 'ordinariness' of this girl, ending the narrative of training with a set of photos that includes a wedding – only the bride is a rather attractive blonde. The subject of the brochure is shown walking into the hospital, wearing her badge and smiling proudly – married to nursing, perhaps? The images are awkwardly situated between photo-realism and comic portrayals of romance, juxtaposing a romanticised ideal of femininity and marriage with the alternative of nursing. On the last page of the brochure, these two positions are reconciled by the text: 'married or not, you'll always be in demand'.

By the mid-1960s, the professionalisers had made sufficient headway within nursing's official structures to seriously challenge the generalists, those in favour of basic training only. The RCN's commitment to education and training was written into its charter; as the professionals began to exert a stronger influence within the RCN, they used this to their advantage. New training courses expanded throughout Britain; tutors began seriously to rival the Matrons as progenitors of occupational ideals as the Matron elite became increasingly frustrated with their position in the new NHS management structures. The grouping together of hospitals to rationalise services had shifted the centre of decision making in the voluntary hospital sector from the hospital board to the Group Secretary; Matrons, accustomed to representing nurses' interests at hospital level, were often excluded from management decisions and lost the direct consultation at managerial level that they had previously enjoyed (Carpenter 1978; White 1986).

Disconcerted at their loss of power, the Matrons agitated for reform, channelling their discontent through the Royal College. This led to the government setting up the Committee on Senior Nursing Staff Structure (Salmon), on which the RCN had a majority voice. The Committee reported in 1965 with recommendations for a modern management structure which it was hoped would restore morale within the profession and provide a clear career structure, the latter acting as an incentive for retaining trained staff in the profession as well as boosting recruitment. It was hoped that the new career structure would attract back to nursing the young middle-class women lost to nursing due to the increasing number of career opportunities becoming available for them, by giving nursing an up-to-date, modern image. The new structure of management created by Salmon had, however, at least one unforeseen effect: it opened the door to career-orientated male nurses.

Recruiting men to general nursing

Between 1950 and 1971, the increase in staff levels in psychiatric hospitals, traditionally an employer of male nursing labour, was less than 5 per cent compared to a 79 per cent increase in general hospitals; general nursing expanded rapidly, while the psychiatric sector grew very little. There is no researched evidence that analyses the influence exerted by senior male nurses on recruitment policies, but by 1968 men were sought actively as potential students of general nursing in the face of continuing attrition by females, although boys leaving school had very little interest in the profession. A survey of English school leavers did not find a single boy who said he intended to take up a career in nursing,[15] but Stones' (1972) survey of male student and pupil nurses found that nursing was attracting job seekers and fresh career men. These trainees saw nursing as a worthwhile, useful job and did not share the popular view of the nurse as a self-sacrificing

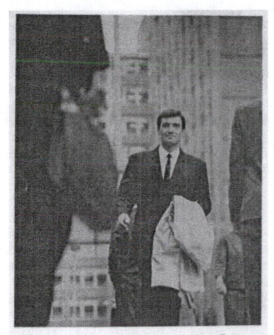

He's stepping out in a career that's different

Figure 3.6 Male recruitment: *He's Stepping out in a Career that's Different*, late 1960s leaflet (Department of Health and Social Security)

paragon. Neither did they see themselves as impersonal nursing technicians. These men were far more career-motivated rather than vocationally orientated in their outlook, and it is the career possibilities in general nursing that are emphasised in the recruitment literature.

By the late 1960s, these publications were working in antithesis to the feminised images of nursing depicted in the literature aimed at women. One brochure depicts a man in a suit, coat over his arm, walking through a high rise cityscape with other men carrying briefcases. '*He's stepping out in a career that's different*', claims the caption heading while never hinting that the difference entails swapping the office and the suit for the ward and a white tunic. The use of a man wearing mufti clearly avoids the issue of how to represent the male nurse at a time when men in general nursing were often considered by many members of the public to be, at the very least, effeminate, more often homosexual. Although there is no mention of this problem of public attitudes in Stones' (1972) study of peer group attitudes to male nurses, the question of sexuality was highly sensitive at the time and must be taken into account in any analysis of images of men in general nursing.

Around the same time, another leaflet was produced that went into the prospects for male nurses in more detail (*Men in Professional Nursing: A Career with Status and Prospects*). Again, the cover avoids any direct association of the word 'nurse' with a nursing image by using clear bold lines of typeface, with the word 'nursing' sandwiched in between them, outlined in orange, virtually filling the page. What catches the eye is the strong black lettering, particularly the word 'men' which is in bold capitals; it takes another look to register 'nursing', by which time the words 'a career with status and prospects' may well have encouraged a job seeker to pick it up. On the first page inside this brochure, three men are pictured in discussion with a female colleague. The text opens with: 'The history of medicine and nursing as the twin arts of healing goes back to ancient times ... today, the part played by men is of vital importance.' The brochure quotes numbers of men in nursing, their distribution in different specialities, and stresses that men hold increasing numbers of the highest positions. Women are marginalised in this brochure both in the text and in the photographs where they are pushed out of the picture to the edges of the frame. There is an emphasis on the technology of nursing care, on the complexity of modern medicine, and on the role that men can play in both general and psychiatric nursing. A clear split in representation is apparent between these two fields of work; general nursing is presented as 'high-tech' curative work, psychiatric nursing as 'caring'.

Brown and Stones found that most of the male trainees they interviewed had actively sought a career in nursing, usually by responding to newspaper advertisements. Many had family contacts with nursing or hospitals and had been members of organisations like the St John Ambulance. They had decided on the basis of their general knowledge that nursing offered attractive career possibilities. Most had humbler origins than female trainees and fewer formal educational qualifications. 'Their image of nursing in general ... is fairly realistic and down to earth. The men did not share the general public's view of the nurse as highly intelligent, dedicated and self-sacrificing. Nursing was a useful and practical skill which could be learned' (Brown and Stones 1973: 114). The men seem to have adopted a functionalist approach to their choice of career at a time when traditional avenues for semi-skilled and skilled training in industry were becoming less available. Unlike their female counterparts, 'it was noticeable that none of the men, when asked about their future career, showed reluctance to be promoted to posts of responsibility which would take them away from bedside nursing – a stumbling block for many women nurses' (*ibid.*).

Men entering nursing for state registration (general) training had fewer formal educational qualifications than their female equivalents; if they had been female, it is possible they might have become state enrolled rather than state registered. The state enrolled nurse, who is invariably female unless he is black, continues to administer 'tender loving care' at the bedside whether he or she is young or old. By 1971, enrolled nurses accounted for one qualified nurse in three, and pupil nurses accounted for nearly a third of all nurses in training. Brown and Stones argue that the female composition of the hospital workplace is a result of specific historical circumstances; they are, of course, right but their analysis is based upon essentialist claims and a rationalist logic that argues for the suitability of nursing as a career for men as it becomes more technical and scientifically based. In their book on the male nurse, Brown and Stones comment that:

> Although there is still a need for the tender loving care traditionally rendered at the bedside by young female nurses there are many other demands on nursing staff. The technical advances required to keep pace with medical developments and increasing specialisation demand types of ability and aptitude which may be found as readily in men as in women . . . Some have argued that men bring a kind of emotional objectivity and technical ability which is ideally suited to the modern world of nursing.
>
> (Brown and Stones 1973: 14)

Caring in general nursing remains firmly within the province of state enrolled nurses and auxiliaries – areas where men were not actively recruited. In both the recruitment literature and the commentary written around male nurses a discourse of professionalism is assumed which values technical nursing work. Never is there a suggestion that the 'tender loving care traditionally rendered at the bedside by young female nurses' could also be done by men. Practical work (the sub-text here is 'dirty' work) and emotional work is left to others – primarily the SEN or the nursing auxiliary, the vast majority of whom are women. Nursing autonomy and professionalisation are increasingly associated with masculine values of emotional objectivity and technical ability, values extensively promoted by an emphasis on academic and scientific education at the expense of learning from the expertise of practising nurses (Salvage 1987a).

Recruitment for men during the early years of the 1970s continued to emphasise the differences between 'high-tech' general nursing and 'caring' psychiatric nursing. A later full colour brochure, *Nursing: A Profession for Men* (1972), attempts to create a high-tech look for nursing through its use of graphics, but the image is undercut by the mid-1970s image of masculinity. A male nurse is depicted on the cover undertaking a nursing task; a square screen border is used to break up the photograph and frame

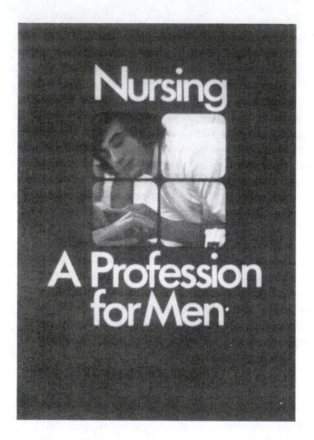

Figure 3.7 Nursing: A Profession for Men, leaflet, 1972 (Department of Health and Social Security)

it, dividing the picture into four sections which creates the effect of a close-up of a man's face as he bends over inspecting a pair of hands. It is undoubtedly the fashionable (for the time) long hair in conjunction with continuing unconsidered prejudices about men in nursing doing 'women's work' that contribute to a possible reading of this image as one of a gay man, an image problem that must have continued to influence male recruitment at this time in spite of a more liberal climate beginning to percolate through British society. In their report Brown and Stones identify several major steps that in their opinion needed to be taken in order to make nursing a more attractive career option for men; significantly, not one of them addresses issues of sexuality.

By 1972, 270,293 (89 per cent) of the 304,834 staff in NHS hospitals in England and Wales were women, including auxiliary nurses and trainees. The male share of the workforce had fallen in real terms from 16 per cent in 1950 to 11 per cent, while numerically the workforce had doubled in size. In spite of their relative decline in numbers, between 1969 and 1972 in all types of hospitals the number of men in the top two grades of Principal Nursing Officer and Chief Nursing Officer increased eightfold, compared to only fivefold for females. (These posts were created as hospitals changed their nursing management systems in line with the recommendations made by the Salmon Report, 1966.) Salvage notes that 'in 1980 almost half of the most senior nursing positions in management, education and various professional organisations, trade unions and statutory bodies concerned with nursing were occupied by men, although in nursing as a whole, men constituted only 10 per cent of the workforce' (1985: 68). The cumulative effects of the male career path in nursing are obvious; men become managers and professionalisers in inverse proportions to their numbers overall. The division of labour in health care, formerly operative between doctors and nurses, has become integral to a division of labour within nursing itself with the rank and file, those who do much of the 'dirty' and emotional work of nursing, remaining overwhelmingly female.

Unsurprisingly, as more men occupied senior positions in nursing, they assumed expert status as managers and educationalists. In spite of a significantly lower educational achievement base than their female equivalents and their comparatively 'lower' class origins, ambitious men were not at all disadvantaged by their gender difference unless they were black: black nurses faced disadvantage and discrimination at every stage of their careers.

Racial divisions: visible differences

It is arguable that the strongest challenge to nursing's image of middle-class white femininity came not from men but from the steady flow of black women entering nursing from the mid-1940s. During this period, many Matrons sought to alleviate their staffing shortages by making use of government policies which saw the training of nurses from the former British colonies as a form of 'overseas aid'. By the time the UK Council for Overseas Student Affairs (UKCOSA) was set up as a charitable body in 1968 to co-ordinate overseas student interests, there were in excess of 17,000 nurses in training from countries outside Britain, a figure inclusive of students, pupils and pupil midwives. One of UKCOSA's first publicly expressed concerns was the position of these nursing 'students', whom they maintained were being used as cheap labour to prop up the NHS. UKCOSA's evidence to the Briggs Committee on Nursing signals an important watershed in the documentation of race relations within the NHS. Until the publication of this report, issues of race and racism had not been raised in the public arena of policy and debate. This is not to say that there had been silence on the issue until this point in time: papers like *Black Voice* had carried articles written by black nurses on the day-to-day discriminatory practices and racist attitudes they constantly confronted in their work (UKCOSA 1971). However, it was only with the publication of the UKCOSA study as a contribution to the evidence placed before the Briggs Committee that any attention began to be paid to these issues in matters of public policy. Given that by this time it was estimated that black labour formed 25 per cent of the nursing workforce overall (Stones 1972) and that black nurses had played a significant role in alleviating the chronic staffing problems faced by the emergent NHS since its inception, the significant absence of their representation in all forms of discourse related to the nursing profession warrants investigation.[16] This invisibility goes beyond the mere fact that images of black nurses were not used in recruitment, although of course this did in the long-term affect the recruitment of British-born black people to nursing (Mr R, personal communication 1992; Torkington 1985). It is not a question of whether these representations equate to the real conditions of life as experienced by the majority of black nurses, but of the framework of imaginary concepts that shape and inform a sense of what the material reality of nursing might, could or should be for black nurses. As long as nursing is presented as white, middle-class and feminine those who do not fit this ideal, even if they are 25 per cent of the nursing workforce, are marginalised as outsiders, unlegitimised and lacking in status. When this figure is added to the 11 per cent of male nurses, the total of nurses who are not white or female is 36 per cent but the image of the nurse in the professional imagination continued to be white and female.

The history of black nurses has remained, until recently, a submerged and largely invisible one, missing from even the 'new' histories of nursing written from the late 1970s on. This is partly because these new histories tend to concentrate on the more distant past, but also because black nurses have not made the kinds of in-roads into the nursing hierarchy that male nurses have achieved, remaining largely as rank and file members of the profession in comparatively low status areas of medical care such as geriatrics and psychiatry. Prior to the Second World War these hospitals, many of them situated on the periphery of large urban conurbations, had relied on immigrant Irish labour but as this pool began to shrink Matrons and administrative officers increasingly turned to what was euphemistically termed the 'New Commonwealth' to supplement local recruitment. Overseas recruits tended to enter the least prestigious areas of nursing and were heavily concentrated in those hospitals that had the most severe recruiting problems. At one stage, a hospital in Essex had a nursing labour force consisting of in excess of 95 per cent of people born overseas in countries ranging from Malaysia to Mauritius and the Caribbean (S. Thompson 1974). This 'co-incidence' of low status work and black skin has implications both in terms of the status of black women in the profession overall and in relation to what becomes known about their situation. Absence from the managerial and professional sectors of the nursing hierarchy has resulted in virtual invisibility, since it is only at this level that research gets done, articles are published and policy debated.

Since so many overseas nurses ended up working in the psychiatric sector, much of the writing about their situation tends to emanate from this field rather than from general nursing. Statistics about overseas nurses were not systematically compiled until the early 1970s, so there is no way of knowing how many overseas students came to Britain to train as nurses, where they trained, what qualifications they achieved and whether they stayed in Britain or returned home. What is known is that most of these students came from Africa, Malaysia and the Caribbean; many came expecting to train as state registered general nurses, the only qualification recognised in their home countries, and found themselves training for state enrolment often in specialities such as psychiatry and mental subnormality – specialities which did not exist at home.[17] These various kinds of training were not apparent to them when they applied to train, and do not seem to have been explained to them on their arrival or subsequently, resulting in many students achieving qualifications that would be of little use to them in their own countries (UKCOSA 1971). In addition, these applicants did not have any notion of the kinds of difficulties they would have to face because of the colour of their skin, a fact that most of the literature in this area tends to ignore.

In a letter to the *Nursing Times*, a student nurse training at an Oxford teaching hospital in 1953 points out that for nursing to be a profession it was essential to have a status hierarchy, since all professions maintain their power through exclusivity. Many overseas nurses started their careers at the bottom of this hierarchy; not only had they been recruited into the least prestigious and least powerful sectors of the profession, but within this sector they tended to be trained for the roll rather than the register. The 25 per cent of the nursing workforce who were black were heavily concentrated in low grades at the bottom, doing physically and emotionally demanding nursing work for the poorest wages. Historical divisions in nursing and the hospital system that were unresolved by nationalisation worked particularly to disadvantage black nurses as they took over the work formerly undertaken by working-class men and women. The seeds of institutional racism sown in the nineteenth-century imperialist project bore a bitter fruit for these trainees; overseas 'aid' supplied a labour force for the work that white Britons no longer wished to do. Neither the work experience nor the qualifications were of use to students who wished to return home after training. It is therefore at the very least euphemistic to describe as 'aid' a practice which had grown in response to a national labour crisis.

The RCN's attitude to the problems of overseas students in the light of UKCOSA's evidence certainly acknowledges this problem, stating that many recruits came expecting to be learners and instead found that they were labourers. They also admitted that many students were channelled into state enrolment, but qualified their position by adding, 'Many of those accepted for training in this country would not meet their own national requirements for acceptance for training. It is believed that steps should be taken to ensure that nursing students from overseas are of a standard comparable to that required of students in this country and that they are reasonably proficient in English' (RCN, evidence to the Committee on Nursing, 1971: para. 62). Although the evidence is sketchy, the facts seem to indicate that the RCN's assumptions are actually just that, statements made without sufficient research to support them. In a study of educational attainment of male overseas recruits, Stones points out that in terms of GCE qualifications at 'O' and 'A' level, overseas men were far superior to their British counterparts although 64 per cent of his sample were rejected from student training. They also had a comparatively higher success rate in examinations for both the register and the roll (Stones 1972). The RCN state in their evidence that one of the main factors affecting the recruitment and retention of trained staff was an 'undue reliance on overseas recruitment'. Stones argues that this was not the case; a GNC wastage study of the period 1957–9 had shown little difference between the wastage rates of student nurses from the UK, Ireland and the Commonwealth. In fact, 'in general and mental training schools Commonwealth students had consistently higher pass rates than students from other countries'. The results of Stones' survey of male psychiatric recruits showed that male overseas students were more stable during training than their British counterparts, with British wastage rates higher in all types of hospital (Stones 1972: 141–4). It is therefore significant that the RCN was seeing overseas nurses as a 'problem' given the history of difficulties experienced by the profession in attracting their 'ideal type' of candidate and retaining these white, middle-class British women after qualification. Could it be that the RCN, unable to come to terms with the changing composition of the nursing workforce, saw increasing numbers of black nurses as a threat to the profession's public image and status?

In her review of the literature on recruitment to and withdrawal from nurse training programmes published in 1969, MacGuire summarised over 60 research projects published since 1940 which have a direct bearing on recruitment (MacGuire 1969). Few include any analysis of overseas students, partly because most of the research was conducted in training schools based in teaching hospitals attached to university medical schools, areas where overseas students rarely trained or worked. They are therefore unrepresented in the research relative to their numbers overall. However, Bannister and Presley's 'Test selection of overseas nursing candidates: A cross validation study' (*Bulletin of the British Psychological Society*, July 1967) concluded that neither the Progressive Matrices Test nor the GNC overseas test 'provided an adequate basis for the selection of overseas candidates' (MacGuire 1969: 134). Their conclusions support earlier reservations expressed by Crookes and French on the 'suitability of using the Progressive Matrices Test with West Indian students' (1961, in *ibid.*: 166). Knight's study on recruitment and wastage of staff amongst 7,435 student and pupil nurses recruited into hospitals in the South East Metropolitan Region between 1961 and 1965 found that students from Eire and overseas had the lowest discontinuation rates (*ibid.*: 178). These studies not only point to the lower attrition levels amongst overseas nurses, but also question the validity of the testing methods that placed so many of them in pupil nurse training programmes.

In the only study of black nurses in MacGuire's literature survey, Martin investigated 'West Indian pupil nurses and their problems in training', interviewing forty-six nurses at a metropolitan geriatric hospital and following up the careers of 95 nurses admitted to the roll in 1958–64. Four-fifths had left the hospital in the first twelve months after enrolment, and few had stayed longer than twelve months. The reasons for this are described as 'attitudinal aggression' through being cast in the role of 'stranger' and the 'unrealistically high expectations' expressed by interviewees who were leaving to become 'proper' nurses by undertaking SRN training (1965, in *ibid.*: 186). Another researcher might have interpreted these results quite differently, pointing out that groups of people, faced with very different situations from those that they had imagined (or were led to believe?), found sufficient strength and solidarity to maintain their self-esteem and to try and improve their situation! This study, like so many of the studies of attrition discussed earlier, tends to emphasise personal characteristics as the principal cause of the problem, rather than examining institutional failure.

Public knowledge of black nurses' experiences of recruitment and training in Britain remains scant. In recent years, attempts have been made to fill in some of the gaps with evidence compiled from oral histories. In *The Heart of the Race: Black Women's Lives in Britain*, Bryan, Dadzie and Scafe have recorded interviews with Caribbean women from all walks of life who found themselves, for one reason or another, in Britain from the early 1950s. They say that in the Caribbean, nursing was (and still is) a highly rated profession, 'respected enough to attract black women already in work to give up their jobs, and come to Britain to train as nurses' (1985: 38). The promise of a better life in England, 'the way they made it sound in the recruitment adverts and broadcasts' (*ibid.*: 24), created a horizon of expectation for many people that was doomed to disappointment. The weather, the cities, food, housing conditions and the unfriendly, racist attitudes of the native population hardly matched the promise of a better life, but once here, few had the resources to leave. Many had to send a proportion of the training allowance home to support relatives and repay the money borrowed to pay the fare. Many trainees, expecting to be students, found themselves on pupil courses with no choice in the matter and no opportunity, because of financial limitations and immigration restrictions, of trying another training institution. Others found themselves as auxiliaries or ward maids, unable to train either because their qualifications were in question, they had failed the GNC test or their English was considered inadequate. Because of their financial situation, many could not afford to leave and had to remain, no matter how unhappy they were. Lee (1976) found as many as 42.6 per cent of his sample fell into this category (quoted in Baxter 1988).

There was no uniformity in the processes of recruitment and selection of candidates. Some trainees wrote to hospitals directly in response to adverts placed in the local paper, or were recruited by hospital representatives (usually the Matron) visiting their home town/country. Others wrote to hospitals where friends were already training, or used agencies, which made all the arrangements at inflated prices. Applications could also be made through the government offices of the home country, which vetted applications and passed them on via the consulate to a British hospital. Others entered Britain on other terms (often as the wife of a student visa holder) and then applied for training. GNC guidelines were used for vetting locally obtained qualifications, which included an English language qualification as part of the minimum requirement, but very few attempts were made to test spoken English before a candidate left her own country. The student, arriving with the expectation of studying for state registration, could find herself placed as an auxiliary or a pupil nurse because her qualifications or her spoken English were judged to be inadequate, and she had failed the GNC test. By this time, she rarely had a choice; she had to accept both the decision and the situation she found herself in.

In 1988, Training in Health and Race produced a campaigning document which argued the case for equal opportunities in nursing. Their survey of the literature pointed out how most of the studies conducted between 1970 and 1980 on overseas trainees emphasise cultural differences when trying to explain the problems experienced by black nurses (Baxter 1988: 18). Baxter points out that it is only in the work of Hicks (1982) that racism emerges as the principal cause of disadvantage and frustration experienced by black nurses, but even here 'there is no analysis of how racism is mediated by the complexities of organisational control, power and social relations' (Baxter 1988: 22). Given the paucity of information Baxter and her colleagues undertook a series of case studies which aimed to make the history of black nurses and their experiences of racism within the NHS more visible. The results are sobering, and indicate something of the personal trauma experienced by many overseas trainees when they arrived in Britain. In addition, Baxter's study reveals the problems experienced by British-born black recruits, some of whom were channelled into SEN training even though they had passed the GNC test. Many found it impossible to transfer to SRN training even after they became state enrolled.

Some nurses clearly felt that it was the prejudices and attitudes of some of their managers that were their biggest obstacle, and that this prejudice existed as much amongst the teaching staff as it did amongst those in administration.

Partly as a result of their parents' experience, many young black school leavers, particularly those with Afro-Caribbean backgrounds, internalised an 'SEN' image of themselves as a 'protection' against the possible indignities of SRN rejection (Baxter 1988: 27–9). Mr R's experience of recruiting trainees in Liverpool in the 1970s supports Baxter's thesis:

> Principal (Divisional) Nursing Officers were not in favour of having 'too many black faces' on the wards – albeit they would rarely admit to it. On the other [hand] as I discovered when talking to school pupils or at careers conventions, the local black pupils had a self-denigrating attitude, in that they did not believe they were 'clever enough', or worse still, that being black they would never be accepted for training at a Liverpool hospital.
>
> (Mr R, personal communication, 1992)

Baxter points out that Asian girls are often discouraged from pursuing nursing as a career by career guidance at school, ostensibly because of the uniform restrictions, whereas well-qualified British-born Afro-Caribbean women still have to combat the stereotypical view that nursing is the most suitable career for them (1988: 29).

Baxter's study highlights the discriminations faced by black nurses at every stage of their careers. Not only did they have more difficulty in being accepted for SRN training, but they then went on to face poor promotion prospects, even though often 'acting up' in senior posts. Those who do find their way into management are often faced with a lack of co-operation from white staff and have to work twice as hard to prove themselves. 'A survey of six health authorities in 1983 revealed that there were no black district nursing officers, only two of the directors of nursing services were black, as were only seven senior nurses' (Baxter, summarising Agbolegbe's (1984) paper 'Fighting the racist disease', 1988: 16). Often, black female managers have to face the double disadvantages of racism and sexism in a working environment increasingly dominated by male managers.

Many of the nurses Baxter interviewed felt considerable pressure to conform to a white image of nursing. This was felt most acutely in relation to management's comments on hairstyle and body image. Assertion of cultural identity through hairstyle, such as wearing plaits, met with considerable opposition even though hair was worn away from the face and off the shoulders, in line with hospital regulations. To quote one of Baxter's interviewees,

Nursing bosses continually make remarks about the unsuitability of a black nurse's physique for the various uniforms that are worn. Throughout a nurse's training, it is stressed that one's appearance is just as important as a skill. Not just any appearance but the one that is acceptable on the ward – that of a 24 year old white nurse.

(Baxter 1988: 56)

This last comment demonstrates how the image of nursing is not just a matter of the content of representation. The image of itself that the nursing profession has presented and promoted is an ideological construct of white femininity that deeply pervades all levels of the profession; it is a framework of ideas, beliefs and attitudes demonstrated in material practices. In trying to assess which factors have contributed to sustaining that practice in the years 1950–75, some conclusions can be drawn. Before I do that, however, it is necessary to examine the conclusions that the Briggs Committee on Nursing reached, since this was the first government body with a specific brief to analyse and comment on the image of nursing.

Image and identity: Briggs and the image of nursing

By the late 1960s, the recruitment problem had not only continued unabated but intensified, along with a growing dissatisfaction throughout all sectors of nursing with levels of pay and working conditions. Nurses' pay by this time had fallen so far behind that of other workers that in some cases hospital domestic and cleaning staff were earning more than the lower grades of nursing staff. The RCN, faced with increasing pressure from members, broke with their anti-political action stance, instigating a major programme of protest now known in nursing history as 'the raise the roof campaign'. In response a Royal Commission was set up by the then Labour government to: 'review the role of the nurse and midwife in hospital and the community and the education and training needed for that role, so that the best use is made of available manpower to meet the needs of an integrated health service' (Briggs 1972).

By 1974, the gains achieved by the 22 per cent pay rise of 1970 had been whittled away by inflation and there was further unrest, this time far more militant in character. Nurses' wages had fallen below those of other skilled female workers like shorthand typists and primary school teachers. For the first time, nurses walked off the wards, demonstrated and marched and worked to rule. Consensus within the profession had broken down. Many nurses joined demonstrations and protests, renewing their demands for a decent wage and an end to split shift duties and twelve-hour working days and nights. Pictures of dissenting nurses marching in protest wearing their nurses' uniforms caused disquiet amongst managers and professional leaders and are largely absent from modern histories of nursing. Baly (1980), for example, dismisses the events as part of a climate of national discontent even though the action secured the largest pay rise of the post-war years and finally gave nurses a degree of parity with other female workers.

The post-war image of nursing proclaimed in 1950s recruitment literature was one of discipline and service. In *Your Chance* (1950), the ambitious working-class girl is hailed by a potentially familiar image associated with adventure and excitement; the brochure promises not only a job, but 'a career with status and prospects', an opportunity to change her social status through training and dedication to duty. This image conveys the strength of the managers in recruiting policy at that time, and the growing commitment amongst senior nurses to recruit enough nurses to staff the newly formed NHS. Its counterpart is the material designed to address a middle-class, grammar school readership produced by the Nursing Recruitment Service, which promises authority and professional autonomy. By the late 1960s, these two polarities are no longer represented in quite the same way. The government literature has divided into training for registration and training for enrolment. The former tends to emphasise the high-tech drama of modern medicine in brochures like *SRN* (1965), with its dramatic use of black and white documentary photography; the latter tends to play on popular fantasies of nursing and femininity such as physical attractiveness, romance and maternal care. Documentary realism is used to attract the professionally inclined (middle-class) reader, whilst discourses of service embedded in a sub-text of romance and motherhood are used to appeal to practical (working-class) girls. Leaflets, on the other hand, tried to appeal to young women across the board, with the result that a variety of approaches were tried, from the innocently inviting appeal of *Nursing* (1966), to the comic cartoon style of *Want to Be a Nurse* (1970), with its play on fashionable hair cuts and large eyes, popularly known at the time as the 'Biba' look.

The recruitment crisis motivated a campaign to persuade trained married nurses to return to work, and older women to take up training for the first time. Much of the appeal to older women was conducted through the pages of popular women's magazines like *Woman* and *Woman's Own*. In *Too Old to Train for Nursing?* (1969), the letter format of personal testimony is used to persuade mature women that training in later life can be both personally and financially rewarding. *Like to be Back in Nursing?* (Leaflet NL 027, 1972) uses the 'makeover' approach common in many women's magazines of the time, where a new make-up regime and a hairdo are seen as the solution to lack of confidence and a poor self-image. This form of masquerade is used in nursing recruitment to emphasise how a return to nursing can be revitalising, creating a new (youthful) lease of life. Soft focus photography and yellow filters are used to accentuate the impression of longing and depression in the picture of the woman on the front of the brochure, while over the page the harder lighting makes

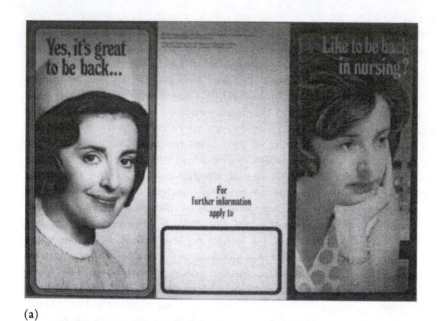

(a)

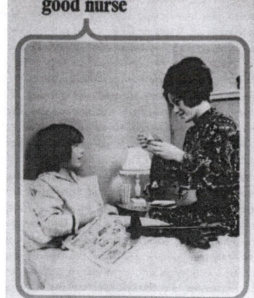

(b)

Figures 3.8(a) and 3.8(b) Targeting the 'redundant' mother: *Like to be Back in Nursing? Yes, it's Great to be Back* (1972) and *You'd Make a Good Nurse* (1973), leaflets (Department of Health and Social Security)

the contrasting colours of hair and make-up stand out brightly against the whiteness of the uniform. The sub-text is, of course, the re-invigoration of the redundant mother, an explicit association used in the 1973 brochure *You'd Make a Good Nurse*, which pictures a woman talking to an older (sick) child on its cover.

By the early 1970s, nursing recruitment for state enrolment had become deeply enmeshed in fictioning an exaggeratedly feminine nursing identity. In *A Girl Like You* (1970), there are clear references in the address of the title to the words of a pop song ('It takes a girl like you to make a dream come true') and in the imagery to contemporary advertisements for cheap make-up such as those used to sell the popular brand 'Outdoor Girl' available in Woolworths at the time. Like its predecessor *Proud Badge of Service* (1966), this brochure emphasises how unexceptional 'Philomena' is, although the use of an unusual Irish name undercuts the 'ordinariness' of the brochure's address. The appeal is still to those who are upwardly aspiring, but in this case good looks and attractiveness (heightened by soft focus photography and low contrast lighting to create a soft, feminine image) are foregrounded against the harsher black and white documentary 'realities of modern hospital life'. The SRN and SEN brochures of the mid-1960s have fused in this 1970s SEN edition; but instead of a sub-text of marriage, romance promises a fun social life and a doctor boyfriend with a sports car, while the drama of working life emphasises the high-tech of the operating theatre. The melodrama of the life and death struggle becomes the *mise-en-scène* for fun and romance, echoing the narrative strategies and realism of hospital soap and the more exotic locations of doctor/nurse romances.

Fiction and reality have apparently fused. The image of nursing promoted by the profession is also the image of the nurse found in many popular fictional narratives. The gradual assimilation of one discourse with the other was a result of a desire to create an imaginary homogeneous community of nurses. The gradual disappearance of images of authority in anything other than teaching roles, while perhaps creating a more friendly picture of hospital work, also lowered the threshold of expectation of those coming into nursing, since individuals were only interpolated as trainees, never as qualified nurses in positions of responsibility. The future, as a qualified nurse, became a distant reality compared to the sense of drama and immediacy created by documentary style photography and the possibilities of fun and romance. The romantic, angelic image of nursing reached its zenith in *A Girl Like You*, but was contradicted publicly by media images of anger and dissatisfaction. This contradiction was of interest to the Briggs Committee.

The Briggs Committee was set up in 1970 'to relieve the [Labour] government's embarrassment over the threat posed by nurses to its prices and incomes policy' (Dingwall *et al.* 1988: 205). This situation is seen by Dingwall as typical of the Labour government of the time which used

Commissions and Departmental Committees to deflect immediate political problems. Rather than quantifying or assessing the effects of any changes that may have been needed for reform, Briggs had to work within the existing manpower and budgetary constraints. Because the committee were unable to consider financial or staffing issues, managerial interests absented themselves from the discussions by arguing that there were no 'resource implications', leaving the field clear for the professionalisers who had a strong base in the RCN.

Dingwall is somewhat dismissive of the report because of its lack of attention to economic and structural reform, but Baly heralds it as a triumph of professional nursing and the RCN. In her view, 'The evidence given by the Royal College of Nursing and contributed to by so many people is worth recalling in order to stress that the impetus for a new philosophy and the need for unified government of the profession came from nurses themselves' (Baly 1980: 322). It is, then, the professionalisers' view of the image of the nurse which is reflected in the Report of the Committee on Nursing, published in 1972. The Briggs Committee devoted a surprising amount of space to the public perception of nursing, examining those aspects of the image of modern nursing which seemed to be historically determined. These were identified and summarised as:

(a) doctor's handmaiden
(b) nurses' fight for their professional status
(c) the class aspect of the vocational ideal
(d) an authoritarian hierarchy created by 'the search for perfection and the attempt to achieve it by discipline'.

References to issues of sexuality, race and gender are disregarded by this historical approach and are not broached by the committee. Briggs considered that these images and ideals were reinforced by mass communications, which look backwards to Victorian Britain and its values as well as forward to an age of integration. Amongst the most influential media images, Briggs singled out books and mass circulation magazines, television series, films and newspapers. Briggs was convinced that these images influence recruitment and 'predetermine attitudes at critical moments in the health history of individuals and families'. There is no mention in the report of pornographic representation, or of the increasing numbers of popular films which in some way questioned or mocked the traditional nursing image.

In an examination of the existent recruitment literature, Briggs commented on the variety of jobs in nursing and midwifery, the emphasis on teamwork rather than individual vocation, and the personalisation of the brochures, dealing with different career profiles and different career aspirations within the profession. The brochure *Something Special*, brought out in 1972, uses a 'take four girls' approach, following the training and careers of four women from very different backgrounds with a range of ages. Significantly, the women are still all white, and there are no equivalent profiles for men, but the separate brochures for training for the register and training for the roll have fused and there is an associated emphasis on teamwork. The emphasis by this time was on the need to care for others in an increasingly complex society; nursing was 'something special' and inwardly rewarding. Briggs saw these changes as recognition by the nursing establishment that they had to change.

The Committee sought the opinion of new recruits to see if there was a gap between the image portrayed in recruitment literature and the experience of training. Answers to the questionnaires suggested that dissat-isfaction with work, hours and shifts was less prevalent than expected, but that nonetheless there was a significant amount of complaint about the drudgery of non-nursing duties and the attitudes and behaviour of nurses themselves (Morton-Williams and Berthoud 1971). Briggs' concluding comment in this part of the report is a salutary one, and it is worth quoting in full since it does point to one of the main themes of this book, that women oppress other women for reasons of power and status:

> After examining together all the criticisms and hopes of improve-ment, we wish to stress that unless sympathetic care within nursing and midwifery administration is shown to nurses and midwives both in training and after they are trained, the wider claims of the profession to rest on individual care will ring hollow. Care starts with the relations between nurses and nurses. So too does sympathetic understanding on which all care is based.
>
> (Command 5115: 38)

The literature on images of nurses pays scant attention to the ways in which women who are nurses think about themselves professionally. In the following chapter, the public and professional images of nursing analysed in these first two chapters are used as a starting point in discussions of nursing identity with women who became nurses between 1950 and 1975. The issue of self-conception is explored here from several angles, using autobiographical writings and case studies. What emerges is a considerably more complex image of nursing identity than that which has emerged so far, but given the disparity of viewpoints solicited, a surprising degree of consensus emerges about what might constitute an ideal self-image, a 'proper nurse'.

4

THE PERSONAL
IMAGINATION

The relationship between the image, a point of view and 'an involvement in the real' problematises any simple tale of the self.
(Probyn 1993: 105)

Autobiographical writings and case studies are used in this chapter to explore the relationship between the self as an image – in the role of nurse – and formations of nursing identity used to image that self. Personal accounts of nursing lives are figured against the ground of public and professional discourses discussed in previous chapters. Several of the studies on recruitment and attrition collated by MacGuire (1969) claim that the image of nursing held by a girl was the most important factor in her self-assessed suitability for training, but there is no indication in these accounts of what image that might have been, or of how young women viewed nurses and nursing during this period.[1] The assumption seems to have been that teenage girls who embraced the romantic notion of serving suffering humanity were those most likely to become nurses, a view confirmed by Miss H, a retired Sister Tutor formerly in charge of nursing recruitment at Liverpool Royal Infirmary throughout much of this period (personal communication, 1992). In these former voluntary hospitals, with their traditional allegiances to religious and charitable institutions, ideals of nursing as a vocation continued to be imbued into young trainees. On the strength of the autobiographies and case studies presented here, however, I will argue that it is highly questionable whether all potential trainees saw themselves (or their new profession) in quite such a romantic or vocational light.

The autobiographical accounts are not intended to map the field of personal recollections about nursing lives, which is a rather vast one and worthy of a study of its own. Rather, they are a sample whose selection has been based on popularity and availability; like the other cultural artifacts discussed in this book, all are or have been widely available, in this case in bookshops and on public library shelves. They are part of the popular discourse on nursing's professional identity, illuminating what it means in day-to-day terms to practise nursing. A principal criterion for selection was that the books should discuss general nursing training and its aftermath between the Second World War and the mid-1970s, irrespective of whether they were published at the time or more recently. All five of those selected have been written by white women trained in British hospitals – as yet there does not seem to be a widely available account of these experiences written by a black nurse. The list of books in chronological order is as follows: Monica Dickens, *One Pair of Feet* (1942),[2] Jane Grant, *Come Hither, Nurse* (1957),[3] Stella Markham, *The Lamp Was Dimmed* (Hale, London, 1975), Lucilla Andrews, *No Time for Romance* (Corgi, London, 1978), Joan Ash, *Catch Me a Nightingale* (Hale, London, 1992). The publishing and reprint dates of these autobiographies roughly correspond with the cyclical popularity of medical melodramas, with peak moments in the late 1950s and early 1960s and a re-emergence in the mid-1970s with the massive popularity of the TV series *Angels*.

Writers of autobiographies tend to be highly motivated individuals who consider that their story is worth telling and that there are sufficient numbers of people interested in the life and/or the lifestyle they are revealing to want to read about it. The nursing autobiographies under consideration divide into two categories: those written by writers who have at some point experienced nursing training and/or practice, but see it as a secondary activity to their writing career (Dickens, Andrews, Grant) and those who have spent their lives as nurses and are writing their memoirs (Ash, Markham). Collectively, they present an image of a generation of women of similar ages becoming nurses; individually, they represent a range of viewpoints on becoming a nurse and nursing's more immediate past.

The study of women's autobiographical writing has tended to become lodged in departments of literature, where there is an emphasis on the works of well-known authors, although autobiographies by working-class and black writers are increasingly on the agenda. In her introduction to an edited collection of writings on women and autobiography, Estelle Jelinek comments that many autobiographies written by women tend to omit references to their working lives, concentrating instead on the domestic and familial (Jelinek 1980: 9). That cannot be said of any of the autobiographies under consideration here; the working self is seen as the core of the autobiographical 'I' whether that self is constructed primarily as a nurse or primarily as a writer. Jelinek argues that women writers rarely reveal painful and intimate memories in spite of claims that autobiography is a self-revelatory and confessional form. That may be true of the autobiographies of famous women, but it is less applicable to these works; Andrews', Ash's and Markham's texts are of interest precisely because they write intimate accounts of their working lives.

Women's autobiographical writing is of significant interest to feminist sociologists and historians, who are less concerned with the aesthetic forms in which experience is mediated and more concerned with the content of that experience as a representation of daily life. The autobiographies I am going to discuss here fall into this latter category. Written as popular narratives of personal experience for an audience of primarily female readers, they contain little of interest to an aesthetician; as social documents, however, they provide insights into the construction of gendered nursing selves, not only in their descriptions of material circumstances but in their attitudes to the processes of professional assimilation. My use of these documents examines Dorothy Smith's (1988b) concept of 'femininity as discourse' and illustrates a commonly cited Marxist axiom, presented here in a somewhat bowdlerised form: that women make their own lives and tell their own life histories, but they do so under conditions not of their own choosing.

The criterion for the selection of the case studies was that the person was likely to tell an untold story, one that official histories of nursing had not yet fully recorded. Among the interviewees are women who were born outside the British Isles, women who came from working-class backgrounds and a woman who discovered and developed her lesbian identity during the process of nursing training. Two case studies of women who left nursing and did not return, either because of domestic responsibilities or because they decided to change their careers, are included, as are two studies of women who arrived in Britain to train as nurses, but spent their working lives as auxiliaries. In research such as this, it is often customary for the informants to remain anonymous.[4] The following introductory notes provide a brief profile of their careers:

- O came to Britain from Ireland to train for general nursing training in Coventry, early 1950s. She now works one night a week on a midwifery unit in Dorset.[5]
- SA undertook general nursing training at a London teaching hospital, early 1950s. She later became a health visitor and marriage guidance counsellor and is currently undertaking further academic study and research.
- V came to Britain from Barbados to train as a general nurse in Kent, early 1950s. She became an auxiliary nurse in a geriatric hospital and has worked as an auxiliary since then primarily caring for the elderly.
- SC attended pre-nursing school prior to general training at a municipal hospital, late 1950s. She worked in casualty and theatre until becoming a district nurse in the early 1970s and is now a university lecturer in district and community nursing.
- G came to Britain from Barbados to train as a general nurse, early 1960s, and found herself in a small, semi-rural hospital in Yorkshire enrolled as a pupil nurse. She upgraded her SEN qualification to SRN in the late 1960s. After eighteen years as a hospital Sister, she has left to work as a practice nurse.
- J undertook general training at a London teaching hospital, mid-1960s. After spending several years as a health visitor, she is now a lecturer and reader in psychology.

- Ly came to Britain from Barbados to complete her schooling and train as a nurse. She commenced pupil nurse training at a municipal hospital in the late 1960s; after working for sixteen years in a special care baby unit she upgraded her qualification to SRN and is now a staff nurse on a surgical ward.
- M came to Britain from Barbados with her partner to train as a nurse in the early 1960s but failed to secure a training place. She started working as an auxiliary in the early 1970s.
- MS started work as a hairdresser but left to undertake general training at a provincial teaching hospital, early 1970s. She became a district nurse, took a degree in sociology and trained as a counsellor and is currently a nurse and student counsellor in a higher education institute.
- Ju began her general training in a provincial teaching hospital, mid-1970s. After a period as a staff nurse in the accident and emergency department she trained as a midwife. She is in the process of leaving nursing for a new career.

Much like other academic research based on qualitative methodologies, my sampling has depended on the willingness and good faith of those who agreed to be interviewed. Ten women donated their time and energy to this project, and I am aware that I have a responsibility to represent their views fairly and objectively. Their accounts are inevitably highly mediated, shaped by the open-ended structure of the interview, the transcription process from spoken to written language and the ways in which I have incorporated their accounts into this research.

Self-image and uniform identities

In the immediate post-war aftermath, the status of the nurse in the public imagination as a 'ministering angel' was at its peak. There are three princi-pal reasons for the high status given to those doing nursing work at this time: one was the introduction of the NHS which, for the first time, enabled medical and nursing services to be freely available to all as of right; the second was a collective memory of nursing care given to the injured, sick and dying in the extreme circumstances of a war in which civilian as well as military casualties had been high; and third, a dependency on good nursing care for surviving 'the crisis' of infectious diseases in the days before the development of effective drug therapies. Until the early 1950s, nurses were imaged primarily as self-sacrificing 'angels' in films and career novels for girls, driven by a vocational zeal that had much in common with a religious calling. The Ministry of Labour promoted a vocational image of nursing as 'a social service' to young women from working-class backgrounds aspiring to middle-class status through marriage or a career. The professionalisers used the Nursing Recruitment Service and the grammar school-based Association of Headmistresses to promote the 'social value' of nursing, playing down the vocational aspect in favour of presenting high-flying career opportunities for those of 'marked ability and high educational standards'. Underlying these recruitment strategies were unconsidered assumptions about the relationship between women of different classes to images and texts. It was presumed that lower middle- and working-class girls were receptive to romantic, emotional appeals to their 'innate' empathetic capacities as potential wives and mothers (an ethics of care), whereas middle-class girls would respond to the (melo)drama of curative medicine and an appeal to their leadership abilities (an ethics of responsibility). The development of the two-tier training system reflected a belief that young working-class women made good practical nurses and should therefore be trained to remain at the bedside, whereas young middle-class women were professional and managerial material; the former would be responsive to an ideology of vocationalism, the latter would ensure that this ideology was maintained in practice. Trainee nurses either absorbed the vocational ethos or treated nursing as a job that had to be done; if they continued to be hospital nurses after qualification, some would undoubtedly wear the veil of vocational idealism. MS described these women as the epitome of the professional nurse:

> 'These nurses were definitely professional women; they would argue that nursing was a vocation and if the salary increased it would attract the wrong type of girl.'

This ethos still pervaded provincial teaching hospitals in the early 1970s.

Becoming a nurse is both a personal and a public process. At the personal level, an individual undertakes a programme of training that enables her to trade her feminine cultural capital, to practise nursing and earn a living from it. At the public level, individuals are schooled to be cognisant of the parameters of the role of the nurse and become licensed as safe practitioners after a prescribed period of education and training mandated by professional organisations and official policy. To become a nurse is to take on both a personal and a public identity, an identity that was symbolised throughout the period of this study by the traditional nurses' uniform. This uniform has historically played a central role in nurses' self-image and is inseparable from the common stereotypes of nursing: the 'ministering angel', the 'battleaxe', the doctor's handmaiden and the sexy nurse. In becoming nurses, young women took on both public fantasies and professional ideals as they donned the uniform. One of the questions that this section of the chapter tries to answer is to what extent individuals who became nurses were aware of these conflicting images of nursing and how they impacted on the process of professional assimilation.

In *Landscape for a Good Woman*, Carolyn Steedman describes her mother's preoccupation with the fashionable 1950s 'New Look' in spite of the prohibitive cost of the clothes for ordinary working women during the years of post-war austerity. A similar preoccupation with fashion and clothes is foregrounded in many of the nursing narratives of the period. In the popular 'career girl' novels, how you look as a nurse, both on and off duty, is of paramount concern. Clothes are used to identify the different types of young women who begin their training in Ealing's (1956) film *The Feminine Touch*. In Jane Grant's autobiographical novel *Come Hither, Nurse* (1957) fashion figures as a mode of resistance and rebellion against the confinement of 1950s femininity; the restraints imposed by senior nurses not only on how the uniform was worn but on off-duty clothes serve as a reminder that the relationship between fashion, femininity and nursing was by no means simple and straightforward.

By the late 1940s, the traditional uniform communicated numerous connotations and associations far removed from the control or influence of professional nursing's orbit, which were a source of both pride and embarrassment to nursing leaders. On the one hand, the uniform was a symbol of nursing's traditional authority and social status; those who wore it were seen to occupy a position of trust and responsibility in society. This was particularly true in the former voluntary hospital sector, where many of the uniforms had changed little since Victorian times. Some of these uniforms bore a direct connection to nursing's religious past; for example, many of the caps worn by trainees were similar to the veils worn by novice nuns, evoking comparable notions of purity, self-abnegation and 'calling' to a higher ideal. J's memories of beginning her training in the mid-1960s at a well-known London teaching hospital recall that even at this time, the religious connotation was still very strong. Etched in her mind is an initial image of religious vocation and duty:

'We were met with what looked like a nun who was in fact our tutor, who was clad in blue and with this sort of cap that came down over her eyebrows and hung down her back. I remember it vividly, it was just like joining some kind of mission really.'

Some uniforms were more reminiscent of Victorian parlourmaids' dresses, with stiff white aprons and starched white collars, frilly hats and thick black stockings. Feminist research has revealed the connections between Victorian female servants and the production of erotic literature and photographic images (Davidoff 1983, Stanley 1984). The uniform has provided a wealth of imagery to feed the pornographic imagination; soft-porn images of scantily dressed nurses showing their brassieres and suspenders (as in the *Carry On* films) are but the tip of an iceberg of submerged pornographic representations featuring nurses.[6] Some uniforms combined the plain apron of domestic service with the lace cap of a lady and the starched Eton collar of the male officer class, displaying the fragmented historical identity of a profession riven by issues of class and status. Young women wearing these uniforms were not only announcing their status as nurses to others, they were literally wearing nursing history, enveloping themselves in the ghosts of nursing's formidable foremothers and their determination to make nursing a respectable profession.

Starched white aprons, high white collars and stiff white hats signify an almost untouchable purity, calling to mind the 'cleanliness is next to godliness' cliche.[7] But nursing as a job necessitates that you come into contact with other people's bodies and their excreta; in many ways, it is a 'dirty' job. Nurses become (over) familiar with the physical bodies of patients who are basically strangers, and as a result of this contact develop knowledge of bodily functions. Such knowledge was still considered unseemly for 'genteel' middle-class young women brought up in the post-war period, whereas working-class girls, judged by middle-class sensibilities and standards, were assumed to be 'closer to nature', more physical and therefore more familiar with (and in need of less protection from) the physical needs and demands of the body.[8] The image of nursing has always tended to embrace both of these feminine stereotypes; on the one hand, an asexualised virginal purity (associated with its religious mission) and on the other a sensual, physical familiarity (associated with working-class servants). In some ways, the uniform was a great leveller, communicating contradictory messages of an untouchable innocence and maternal power. Class issues tended to be subsumed by the uniform; anyone wearing it was open to being seen not only as a virtuous 'angel' but also as a sexualised, worldly-wise female: a tantalising combination of ingenuousness and prurience could be invoked by a patient no matter who was wearing the uniform. This ambiguity lies at the heart of nursing's public image, in spite of changes to the uniform and a greater acceptance of male nurses from patients of both sexes.[9]

Most nurses have had to cope with this ambiguity at some point in their working lives, which can take the form of anything from good humoured quipping from primarily male patients through to blatant sexual harassment (Ash 1992, Lawler 1991). Jocelyn Lawler considers that sexuality is a pervasive aspect of heterosexual social life; the lack of (reported) sexual harassment of staff working in same-sex situations is at least partly due to codes of containment in lesbian and gay sub-culture which define specific places of acceptable sexual expression (Lawler 1991: 213). The attitudes of female patients to female nurses are more difficult to determine; the lack of research in this area tends to suggest a continuing 'taken for grantedness' in encounters between same-sex nurses and patients. Lawler (1991), for example, focuses on male patients and female nurses in her detailed account of how nurses manage the bodies of others, although she does mention male nurse/ male patient encounters. Markham recalls one instance where a female patient deemed to have an 'unnatural' sexual lust harassed female nurses and made them wary of her; this is the only description of a lesbian patient in the texts examined. There are no images of lesbianism or same-sex relationships between nursing staff.

Ju became aware of her lesbian identity during her training when she met and fell in love with a woman in her cohort:

> 'I wasn't even aware really that I was a lesbian then . . . I decided to leave after I'd finished training, not permanently but I was going to go to Greece for a few months . . . and I decided I was in love with Louise . . . I decided I would only stay if I could get a job in Casualty 'cause that was the only thing I was prepared to do . . . there was a nursing officer who worked in Casualty exclusively and she liked me, she was a dyke and she liked me and she said straight away "yes, there's a job here if you want it"' so I stayed.'

I have found no documented accounts of the experiences of women who share same-sex preferences in British nursing, perhaps because lesbians could pursue professional lives that bore all the hallmarks of feminine respectability without fear of discrimination as long as their private lives remained hidden.[10]

Amongst the nurses interviewed for this project, opinions varied considerably about the degree to which they were either regarded as untouchable 'angels' or subjected to various forms of sexual harassment. O, who started her training in the early 1950s, commented as follows:

> 'People, especially Coventry people, held the nurses in great esteem and respected them and looked up to the trained staff especially and I thought, oh yes, one day I'll be there in that position.'

This experience seems close to that of Lucilla Andrews, who trained as a nurse in war-time Britain and talks only of the praise and respect nurses received from the general public. On the other hand, SA, thinking about her training at a London teaching hospital in the early 1950s, commented:

> 'I never quite established how it was that when you were out, men always seemed to know that you were a nurse, whether you stunk of disinfectant or what. You were either an easy lay or an angel, one or the other.'

SC trained at a large municipal hospital in the late 1950s. She pointed out that there was a great division amongst trainees between 'party goers' and 'save souls'. This distinction did not mean that the former had loose morals or that the latter were particularly religious, but it did mean that 'party goers' bore the brunt of being branded 'easy lays', whereas 'save souls' tended not to socialise.[11] These images were still circulating in the 1970s. MS knew that nurses had a 'bad reputation' when she applied to do her training at the local teaching hospital:

> 'There was a slag image, but we were above that, I didn't feel tainted by that.'

It is interesting to note that SA, insecure in her social status, felt 'tainted' by the whore image (as I did myself), whereas MS, secure in her middle-class identity, felt completely immune from it.

Whoever wore a nurses' uniform became a personification of angel/sexy nurse stereotypes, a specific variation of the virgin/whore dichotomy. These binary oppositions were ascribed to nurses somewhat indiscriminately, irrespective of class background or the status of the hospitals that they worked in. To become a nurse was to wear a sign of public service to the community, with associated connotations for some of an underlying liberal maternalistic ethos; on the other hand, nurses evoked personal fantasies of erotic sexuality embedded in the public imagination. An individual nurse could be seen as any (and sometimes all) of the spectrum of illusions ranging from self-sacrificing angel, through visions of hard work and authoritarian control, to fantasies of carnal knowledge and sexual voracity.

One way that the nursing profession has tried to overcome and change these images is through modernising the uniform. Until the late 1960s, change mostly consisted of modifications in dress fabric, length and design; then a slow programme of national reform began. In practice, nurses have always tended to modify their uniforms to suit the style of the day by altering small but significant details; for instance, folding hats in more stylish modes, wearing non-regulation shoes and altering the width of their belts, but this was fairly strictly controlled by peer group pressure to conform to professional ideals:

> 'They were very, very strict . . . I don't think we dared mess around with the uniform. What we used to do of course was to pinch our waist in so that we could hardly breathe, it was obviously important that we had this sort of hour-glass look' (SC).

> '[The uniform] had to be 13 inches off the ground and we had these big hats, all stiff and starchy, black stockings and black shoes. You wouldn't go round with dirty shoes, they were very particular, very strict' (O).

Several nurses commented on how uncomfortable these uniforms were, and how the stiff starched collars rubbed the neck:

'Very uncomfortable, it was like wearing mattress covers ... it wasn't an attractive uniform' (J).

These nurses claimed that, in spite of its problems, the traditional uniform did have a use, and it is perhaps this aspect that has been least taken into account by critics such as Salvage (1987a). For the individual wearing it, the uniform was a crucial interface between a vulnerable private self and the public world of the hospital with its cryptic language and rituals. In this sense, its protective function went beyond the mere practicalities of looking clean; for the novice nurse, it conferred authority and status and gave her the initial confidence needed to approach strangers and carry out nursing duties:

'In those days the nursing uniform was something to wear ... so that when you put those on you know, you feel quite important really ...' (Ly).

'It was obviously quite important to me as a young woman, as a young girl to be wearing a uniform ... we were very, very proud; it was all part of the rites of passage' (SC).

'It felt brilliant' (G).

'I just assumed an identity that was quite important for me, that made me feel quite strong and powerful ... with my uniform on at work, it gave me a lot of confidence, yes' (Ju).

As well as conferring authority and status, the uniform had a protective function, enabling the wearer to perform personal acts of body work on complete strangers. It was both a tangible and a metaphorical barrier, functioning in a similar way to the bar counter that separated Victorian barmaids from their (often lascivious) customers (Bailey 1990). The nurses in this study felt that the traditional uniform was in some sense an integral part of their identity as nurses, for all the criticisms they might have of it.

Perhaps this is unsurprising; all but one worked in hospitals in the days when various forms of the traditional uniform were still worn whether you entered the profession as a cadet nurse, a student, a pupil or an auxiliary. In one way, the uniform was a great leveller. As long as you wore it, to the patients you were a nurse, no matter what hierarchical status values were professionally attached to differences in caps, belts and dresses. In another way though, the uniform was a great divider, keeping the different grades of nurse strictly apart and maintaining rigid hierarchical boundaries within the profession.

The uniform has been on and off the nursing policy agenda since the Briggs Report in 1972, when it was pointed out that the image projected to the public was in urgent need of modernisation. The introduction of the national uniform for nurses in the wake of this report became a bone of contention amongst nurses. In her autobiography, Joan Ash describes her return to nursing in the mid-1970s after a long absence spent bringing up her family. Her biggest shock was not the modernisation of treatment and nursing services, but the fact that the nurses were all wearing 'Jeyes cloths'. Instead of finding nurses, Ash felt she had landed amongst a group of Marks and Spencers shop assistants and that 'Without the linen aprons, the familiar figure of the nurse had faded into history' (1992: 58). J expressed a similar feeling even though she was critical of the uniform she had to wear as a trainee:

> 'The national uniform probably did more for lowering the self-esteem of nurses than any other single act. I think how can people feel good about themselves when they're forced to put all shapes and sizes into such ridiculous sorts of uniform . . . it makes you feel not valued, and I think nurses have gone through quite a long period of not feeling terribly well valued.'

This sense of not feeling valued is clearly felt by Ly:

> 'These days, [the nurses' uniform] don't really mean anything. It's horrible now – the girls in Littlewoods dress better than nurses today. There's not much pride in it.'

O feels that the loss of the traditional uniform is part of a much broader decline of the status of the nurse and nursing in society:

> 'Put that uniform on and you were a nurse. If a policeman puts the uniform on, you'd expect him to be a policeman. That's what everyone thinks, you know, and now we're going to lose the lot. We're going to lose our hats and aprons. I think everything is going.'

This is tied in with a sense that the public sees nurses very differently today, something that Ash dwells on at considerable length. In the post-war period, the working-class women surveyed in the National Public Opinion Poll (1966) tended to bestow nurses with an 'angel' image, but middle-class women viewed them more as a specialised type of servant – a view shared by those who defined nursing and domestic work as virtually analogous in the 1949 Nurses Act. Lucilla Andrews comments on how working-class female patients often managed their stay in hospital through a sense of camaraderie, sharing good humoured bawdy jokes and banter that she rarely understood (Andrews 1978: 113). My own memory is that many nurses actually disliked nursing women, particularly on the private wards where the middle-class patients were often considered 'over-demanding'; but much of this antipathy evolved from the burdensome nature of the workload on the female wards – the endless round of bedpans and heavy lifting.[12] Some female patients recognised nursing as hard work, but others expected it as a right, as part of the hospital service.

Post-1970s, the public have a much less romanticised image of nurses; they are no longer respected authority figures or comforting pseudo-mothers. Ash's autobiography is peppered with descriptions of patients physically assaulting the nursing staff, assaults that occur more frequently as her account moves into the 1980s. This loss of respect and value is seen by some nurses as a direct result of an increasingly militant attitude which puts professional and personal needs before those of the patients. Markham, for example, writing in the mid-1970s, is highly critical of professional preoccupations with pay and conditions of service, and sees them as primarily responsible for changing public attitudes towards nursing:

> I am grateful for the better salary and the better conditions, but I think that a lot has been lost in the gaining of these, and that we must accept that there is something intangible in the old fash-ioned word 'vocation'.
>
> (1975: 167)

In contrast to this view, Ash displays a determined militancy against a bureaucratic system which, she feels, has systematically destroyed her profes-sional values and beliefs. Entering the profession from a strict Christian upbringing, Ash became a vocationalist after her initial training in the 1940s when she 'fell passionately in love with nursing'. By the 1980s, however, her militancy is not one that sits easily with traditional ideas of vocation-alism and self-sacrifice although her fight is in part about protecting these ideas and values from further erosion.

Others view the changes in public attitudes with more mixed feelings; for these nurses, the loss of professional aura is seen as the direct result of a public becoming more informed and educated on health and medical matters. Higher standards of general education and specifically more infor-mation about their own bodies has accompanied a general loss of belief in the miraculous powers of modern medicine that characterised 1950s society. As O regretfully stated,

> 'There's no secrecy, everybody knows what we do and there's no barriers anymore . . .'

For Ly, this change in attitude has practical implications in administering treatments because patients have the right to say 'no':

'I felt the attitudes then were a lot different to what they are now ... they had a lot more respect for you and whatever you say, they would do it, they felt that you know best. I suppose they put all their trust in you really ... they're a lot more educated these days. They ask more questions, they know a lot more about their body.'

Whether these changes in public attitude towards nurses can be attributed primarily to an increase in people's knowledge about their bodies, or to consumerist lobbies that have fought for more rights for patients in health care practices (a movement that culminated in the Patients Charter of 1992) is not a question that can be answered here. The question of status is, however, of vital importance in the new market economy of health care in terms of nursing's ability to continue to be able to differentiate its services from those of other para-medical professional groups. It is also of critical importance in recruiting young women and men into the profession, for if nursing's professional status has low public value, those seeking a satisfying career will be more inclined to enter fields where the rewards, in both status and financial terms, are greater.

Knowing your place: hierarchy, status and the self

By the early 1950s, general nursing had become institutionally hegemonic: state registration as a general nurse became the main portal of entry to all careers in nursing, the gateway to professional status and a wide variety of further qualifications in specialised fields. Other trainings, such as fever nursing or sick children's nursing, began to be seen as specialised additional qualifications, although it was still possible to practise in these areas without a general nursing qualification. There continued to be an acute shortage of people who wanted to do nursing work; the NHS increased the demand for nurses, with the result that the recruitment net was widened to find new sources of labour. One of the new initiatives was the establishment of pre-nursing schools attached to the new secondary modern schools, as well as recruiting more candidates from nursing's traditional pool of immigrant labour, Ireland, and extending recruitment drives to the 'New Commonwealth'. All the interviewees wanted, at some point in their lives, to become state registered general nurses, although, for a range of reasons, not all of them achieved their ambitions. Of the autobiographical writers, only Dickens withdrew from training; the rest became qualified general nurses, but only Ash and Markham worked as nurses for long periods of their lives.

Given that there was an acute labour shortage in nursing, relying on the vocational image was clearly an insufficient answer to the problem of attracting the large numbers of young women that were needed to staff the wards. Nursing leaders who supported the management ethos of the new NHS used a variety of popular fictional images of the nurse to appeal to young working-class women, in contrast to the more traditional 'lady of the lamp' ethos used by the professionalisers.

Monica Dickens was probably the single most influential portrayer of professional nursing identity throughout the 1940s and 1950s. Her auto-biographical novel *One Pair of Feet* (1942), based on her experience as a first year nursing trainee, led to a film adaptation *The Lamp Still Burns* (1943) and to co-scriptwriting a nursing recruitment feature film commissioned by the Crown Film Unit for the Ministry of Information, *Life in Her Hands* (1951). Dickens had the support of nurse leaders in the influential London teaching hospitals as well as the Ministry of Health. Her work was popular and found a wide and appreciative audience perhaps because, as *The Listener* commented in a quote published on the book cover, 'Miss Dickens succeeds, almost in spite of herself, in conveying the essential nobility of the profession and the supreme satisfaction of a life saved' (Penguin 1957 edition). The comment 'in spite of herself' succinctly summarises Dickens' view of the nursing profession. Although she admires the espoused values of service, self-sacrifice and dedication to a higher ideal, she finds nurses themselves a rather dull and uninspiring group of women, riven by petty snobberies and class discrimination. A great-granddaughter of the author Charles Dickens, Monica was privately educated and presented at court in 1935. She therefore occupied a markedly different social position in English society from the majority of women who were nurses in war-time Britain. Her sardonic attitude towards many of her nursing colleagues distinctly conveys this sense of class difference. The text is littered with references to their aspirations 'to set [themselves] on a higher plain than their fellows' (1957: 117), a form of snobbery which Dickens, from her secure position in the upper echelons of the social hierarchy, considered 'odious'. Although she mocks the attitudes of those in her peer group who objected to being bossed about by 'uneducated women with no breeding' (1957: 79), she finds the airs and graces adopted by those of a lower class than herself amusing, especially given the menial, servicing nature of much of their work. Commenting on hospital etiquette at this time she says, 'I was always dropping bricks and addressing people as equals' (1957: 33). Her writing conveys an image of a confident and articulate young woman whose difficulties in coping with the servile nature of the work she had to do were emphasised by her low status in the hospital hierarchy. She wryly comments near the beginning of the book: 'Several people had told me that they tried to resist the hospital system at first and had ideas about revolutionising the whole thing. But you can't; it's too big and too rooted' (1957: 36).

To anyone reading this autobiographical novel in the 1990s, Dickens' achievement is one of being able to convey the mindset of a young upper middle-class woman in early 1940s Britain. The desire to explore and write about the lives of women from different backgrounds to herself using methods of participant observation has similarities with the work of her contemporary, George Orwell. These war-time ethnographic writers had much in common with their Victorian literary predecessors such as Charles Dickens and Charles Kingsley – a desire not only to reveal social injustice by informing and educating the reading public, but also a commercial incentive to entertain and amuse. Monica Dickens, however, lacks the radical liberal humanist edge of Orwell; at times her satire serves only to mock the women she observes, without proffering any insight, deeper questioning or analysis into either their institutional positions as female health workers, or the formation of their subjected gender positions as self-sacrificing carers of the sick. Dickens describes a series of possible options for working-class women called up for public service in war-time Britain – in the services, the land army, and the auxiliary fire service, all of which, apart from nursing, she claims to have rejected because of the hard physical labour involved. Opportunities for upper- and middle-class women in war work, such as the Women's Royal Voluntary Service, she dismisses as essentially small-minded. She claims that she chose nursing not only because 'It's one of those adolescent phases like wanting to be a nun', but because she saw Madeleine Carroll in *Vigil in the Night* (1940) at the cinema: 'I was going to be a nurse in a pure white halo cap, and glide swiftly about with oxygen cylinders and, if necessary, give my life for a patient' (1957: 9). Dickens' irony is aimed here at the sentimentality of nursing's vocational ideal and its melodramatic presentation, as well as the tastes of the female cinema audience. On the one hand, she distances herself from this ideal through the implicit critique of her derision; on the other, there is a wry admission that there is something noble about living life in the service of a higher ideal. While she emphasises her awareness of popular forms and, as a 'middle-brow' writer of literature, her own critical distance from them, she also acknowledges the powerful emotive forces generated by working in life and death situations: emotions which popular melodramatic forms can so aptly convey.[13]

   This critical, ironic stance does affect how Dickens' account of becoming a nurse can be interpreted. Her detached, derisive position can be read as a distrust of images that play upon an emotional need to be needed; her middle-class sense of her own self-worth makes her aware that exhortations to women to devote themselves to others can be exploitative, especially in war-time. Dickens was aware of contemporary feminist arguments for equal rights in employment; her comments about the wages, working conditions and the need for unionisation amongst nurses show a sympathy with the plight of working women, although she explicitly refuses to align herself publicly with a feminist critique of conditions. Her deep suspicion of the process of institutional assimilation in nursing comes from a liberal fear of conformity as a threat to individual freedom and personal autonomy. The insularity and routine of much of hospital life changes the self because nurses are trained to obey a set of institutional rules and behavioural regulations, not to use their initiative or express an opinion. Unambitious conversation and the 'unsubtle, lavatorial humour' make Dickens feel dull and inadequate in other social circles (1957: 203). Nurses were not expected to take an interest in the outside world and nor did the outside world, she claims, expect nurses to be interested in outside events (1957: 42). They were regarded, by and large, as 'a race of screaming bores' (1957: 95).

It is perhaps not so much that Dickens disliked nursing work *per se*, but the rigid, hierarchical structures in which that work took place; almost in spite of herself, Dickens does find nursing fascinating and in a way fulfilling. The personal drama of facing her own fears and prejudices is conveyed in her accounts of life and death situations. Although her descriptions of patients, similarly to her descriptions of the nursing staff, tend towards a caricature of 'working-classness', she is aware of patients as people and of a system of health care that perpetuated anxiety and distress amongst patients because of its refusal to share knowledge with them. She is able to discriminate between those Sisters who ran their wards in an atmosphere of care and concern and those who created mini 'totalitarian states', treating nurses and patients alike as mindless imbeciles.

In the films that Dickens scripted this more positive attitude is foregrounded, and nursing is portrayed as a worthy career for their leading protagonists, young middle-class women. Given, however, that the film audience throughout this period tended to consist of women from working- and lower middle-class backgrounds – nursing's traditional source of labour – it can be argued that the melodramatic aspects of the films were presumed to appeal to the romantic, sentimental emotions of the female audience. At this time, there was widespread general agreement on the political left and the right about the susceptibility of women (and by implication, this meant lower-class rather than middle-class women) to manipulation through mass cultural forms.[14] Dickens seems to have been aware of these theories, demonstrated in the ironic parody of her own experiences of becoming a nurse and the critical distance she maintains from her own emotional responses to nursing work.

Of the five autobiographies used in this study, it is Dickens' that is closest to Jelinek's (1980) assessment of female autobiographers. Jelinek claims that women writers are unlikely to reveal painful and intimate memories; intense feelings of love and hate, fear, the disclosure of explicit sexual encounters or the detailing of painful psychological experiences are generally left out (Jelinek 1980: 9). Women, according to Jelinek, generally write in a straightforward and objective manner about their girlhood and adult experiences; they also write obliquely, elliptically or humorously in order to camouflage their feelings. In *Come Hither, Nurse* (Jane Grant, 1957) it

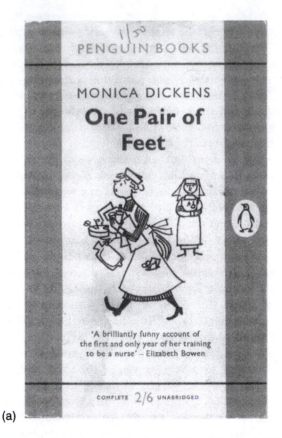

(a)

Figure 4.1(a) Cover, *One Pair of Feet*, Monica Dickens (Penguin Books, 1957)

seems far more plausible that the author has adopted an elliptical or humorous mode in order that her book will sell rather than to hide her feelings. Published at the same time as Richard Gordon's highly popular *Doctor* books, it is likely that Grant was encouraged by her publishers to adopt a similar lightness of tone in the interests of commercial success, just as Andrews was encouraged to write medical romances rather than serious novels.[15] Contemporary critics certainly picked up the similarity to Gordon, comparing Grant rather favourably to Monica Dickens. Reading her text today, the most striking similarity is not to either of these writers but to Sheila Mackay Russell's account of her training in the United States, *The Lamp is Heavy*, adapted by Ealing films to make *The Feminine Touch* (1956). Like the nurses in this film, Grant's nurses spend much of their time observing and caring for the male medical staff rather than their patients. Doctors are supplied with constant cups of tea, sandwiches and patients' food stolen from the fridge. As well as being nurtured by this constant

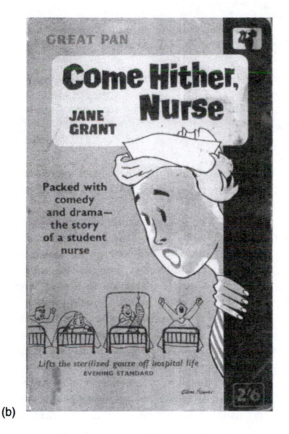

(b)

Figure 4.1(b) Cover, *Come Hither, Nurse,* Jane Grant (Pan Books, 1959)

supply of food and drink by the nursing staff, doctors have their shoes cleaned, their socks washed and numerous other little chores done for them. The image of the nurse as doctors' handmaiden reaches its zenith in this account; nurses no longer administer tender loving care to sick patients, but serve medical men with a passionate zeal. The handmaiden is constructed here as a variation of the ministering angel, with doctors supplanting patients as the objects of selfless devotion.

The text, however, reveals some interesting observations on the doctor/nurse relationship. Towards the end of the book, Jane is in her third year of training and has begun to notice that some of her nursing superiors know considerably more than the medical staff. Aside comments in the text begin to point out how doctors use nurses' experience of problem solving to their own advantage, acting as if they had thought of the proffered solution themselves. The following extract is one of some half a dozen such exchanges in the text:

Totally disregarding the gowns and masks we had put out for them, doctors and students started looking at and discussing the X-ray photograph of the man's jaw. It was obviously going to be a tricky job.

'Why don't you use the magnet, boy?' said Daisy [the night Sister] to the Registrar.

'Yes, we could do', said the Registrar, as if the idea had already occurred to him (which it hadn't).

(1957: 109)

These exchanges bear a striking resemblance to those later observed by ethnographic researchers in participant observation studies of nurse/doctor working relationships.[16]

Grant, like Dickens, addresses her text to the middle-brow market. She is writing for an educated readership who need little explanation about medical procedures or explication of medical terminology or words with Latin prefixes. She speaks as one middle-class person to another, commenting on the habits of her working-class patients as if they were a quaint species of being from a different race or breed. Female patients are regarded as more depressed and sorry for themselves than the men, who are considered much more fun to nurse and better at being patients. Although Grant does not make a direct connection between nurses of lower social status and the 'empty headed gigglers' she dismisses on several occasions, the implication throughout is that there is some sort of connection between class and intelligence. When it comes to her descriptions of the medical staff, however, no such assumptions are made; there are numerous references to thick and stupid doctors who are not very good at their jobs.

Grant makes few references to general attitudes to nursing, other than how it was regarded by friends and relatives as hard work. Nor are there any references to issues of sexuality, apart from having to deal with sexual innuendoes from male patients. Wearing clothes that were considered 'tarty' was definitely frowned on, and results in one of Grant's peer group being asked by the Matron to change her off-duty clothes. Detail about nursing work is rather thin, unless it involves a medical procedure with a doctor present and the opportunity for a romantic encounter. Considerable effort is spent in describing the different ways Jane and her friends manage to procure doctor boyfriends and husbands for themselves; the book is really an adult version of *Sue Barton: Student Nurse* with the emphasis on the rituals of courting itself, rather than preparing for the event of courting through concentrating on the details of clothes and make-up.

The handmaiden image that Grant describes stands in stark contrast to accounts by the interviewees, several of whom pointed out that although ostensibly organised around the care of sick people, hospitals are in fact organised around the work schedules of medical men, whose tasks of diagnosis and prescription are given precedence over the nursing tasks of treatment and care. Although nurses are responsible for day-to-day observations, delivery of treatments and care of patients, their role is circumscribed by medical priorities. In Britain – within the NHS at least – their position in the hospital hierarchy at this time was a somewhat ambiguous one because they were employed by the health authority rather than by doctors, either directly or indirectly. The onus of responsibility fell on nursing management; for most nurses, contact with doctors was fairly minimal:

'It was our job to make sure the patients were kept quiet and the beds spick and span while the doctors were going round – we had very little contact' (J).

'We were separated from the doctors, and not encouraged to socialise. We even had our own eating place' (MS).

Training and status

Amongst the interviewees who began their nursing training in the 1950s, none remembered reading Dickens or Grant, or seeing the films, but they did have clear memories of why they had taken up nursing as a job or career, which hospitals they had trained at and why, and how those hospitals had their own particular methods for instilling their own interpretation of professional nursing values into new recruits. In response to a question about their class status, most of the women claim working- and lower middle-class origins which they now feel varying degrees of distance from, seeing class identities as somewhat fluid; only two interviewees claimed a middle-class position based on their fathers' status. Class consciousness was an issue for those who trained in London teaching hospitals; only two other interviewees expressed strong feelings about nursing's class status.

SA came from a fairly typical upwardly mobile lower middle-class family: her father was a policeman, her mother had trained as a teacher. She had no idea that such a background would make her feel inadequate when she commenced her training in the early 1950s at one of the most prestigious London teaching hospitals:

'I was aware (which hadn't occurred to me until I got there) that I wasn't quite up to it. An awful lot of them were the daughters of doctors ... they were definitely middle-class, which I don't think I was.'

For SA's family, acceptance for training at a London teaching hospital was, by implication, an acceptance of their own upwardly mobile social status, a sign that they had in some sense made it, and crossed an invisible barrier in 1950s society. SA's father's response, which she remembers because it angered her at the time, was that she only had a place because he was a police superintendent, not because of any intrinsic merits she herself possessed. It was his efforts and his career success, not SA's success in the education system, which he saw as the most significant factor in her achievement. For upwardly mobile families in the 1950s, training at a London teaching hospital had a resonance that still echoes faintly today, particularly amongst the older generation. These hospitals were given high status by the general public in part because of their long established charitable associations and religious heritage, but also because of their growing visibility in television medical documentaries as pioneers of new medical miracles. The training schools had created a reputation based not only on their historical connections and the quality of their nursing care but on the social status of their recruits. J's family were of the opinion that if you were going to train as a nurse, you wanted the best training available, and that was to be found in a London teaching hospital.

By the mid-1960s, the class status of entrants to the London teaching hospitals was beginning to change, according to J:

> 'Everybody thought everybody else was going to be far more superior, so everybody adopted terribly posh accents until we suddenly realised that Sally's father was a milkman, and somebody else's father was a postman, and actually we all came from working-class backgrounds, the majority of us, except for two girls who stood out whose fathers were in the RAF. They really didn't mix well with the rest of us; to be honest, we've lost track of them.'

Nicknamed 'the lady apprentices' by their contemporaries, the nurses who trained at the core hospitals in the London teaching hospital group (primarily Guys, St Thomas's, St Bartholomews (Barts), the Westminster, Kings College and the London) were often seen by other nurses as snobbish, 'stand offish' and elitist.[17] Commenting on the awareness between nurses of this internal hierarchy, and referring to the time she worked at Poole General, where the Matron favoured employing nurses trained at Barts, SC pointed out how you could always tell a Barts nurse by her (superior) attitude. J was aware of how this sense of professional superiority had permeated her training:

> 'Barts had a very strong image of what a Barts nurse was, and at the end of PTS [Preliminary Training School] they actually sent away one girl because she wasn't "Barts material".'

Nightingale's influence on the training and education of nurses spread far beyond the London teaching hospitals. Many of those she trained took to reforming nursing and its workforce with a missionary zeal, particularly in the former workhouses and municipal hospitals. As Gamarnikow (1991) has pointed out, Nightingale equated nursing training with learning to be a 'good woman', an idea that appealed to the parents of upwardly mobile, 'respectable' working-class females who could no longer expect to spend their lives in service. In schools of nursing strongly influenced by Nightingale's teachings, the ethos of traditionalism with its vocationalist overtones of self-sacrifice and duty to the patient counteracted the modernising forces of Fordist managerial strategies and unionisation of the workforce. SC describes a training that seems very little different from that experienced by SA and J, although SC emphasises the role played by tradition in her professional assimilation to a greater extent than SA and J. It is difficult to assess whether this emphasis comes from her recent feminist insights into the role of training in maintaining servile feminine role models, or whether the school itself maintained a more traditional ethos than the London teaching hospitals – a reverse form of snobbery.

Unlike SA and J, SC did not have parents who were upwardly mobile themselves. Like many working-class children in the 1950s, she attended a neighbourhood secondary modern school. From there at the age of 15 she took a two-year pre-nursing course run in association with the local municipal hospital, and then worked as a nursing cadet, finally training in the same place. If it had not been for her father's persistence, SC would not have realised her nursing ambitions as she was told that she was too short to become a nurse; popular knowledge of the Nightingale myth, in this case, enabled her father to challenge official dictates:

> 'My father was quite cross; his attitude was to dismiss the official-
> dom ... Florence Nightingale was less than five foot tall ... so
> he sat down and wrote to the local education authority saying that
> if his daughter wanted to be a nurse, her height shouldn't be a
> reason to stop her.'

For SC, becoming a nurse was charged with the magnetism of middle-classness. She describes her nursing ambitions as a mixture of fascination and aspiration – fascination with the trappings of authority that nursing carried, and an aspiration to attain the middle-class lifestyle it seemed to promise. She recalls how she avidly read *The Lady* in an attempt to learn about the mores and values of middle-class femininity. SC's testimony struck strong chords with my own memories, where voice training, learning about art and literature and changing our style of dress were integral to a self-improvement programme designed to address our internalised inferiority as nursing students on the periphery of a university student body.

SA experienced quite a different trajectory from SC; she passed the 'eleven plus' examination and became one of the first scholarship girls to enter the local grammar school. She remembers that her first encounter with class difference was at this school, where her best friend was barred from speaking to her own mother because she was a dinner lady, 'and it wasn't done to speak to people like that'. Although she was an avid reader of the *Sue Barton* books, SA feels it unlikely they had any impact on her decision to become a nurse. The nursing image SA had at the forefront of her mind during the interview was based on hospital admission as a child; the image is one of strict authoritarian femininity with very tall, very straightlaced, stern women caring for her. She became a nurse because of a lack of other available career options:

> 'I really think it was just an acceptable thing to do ... I didn't really want to be a nurse, not initially anyway ... I wanted to go to university, but I was told I wasn't brainy enough which was possibly true.'

SA claims she didn't think about it very much; nursing was just an accepted career choice. She went to visit a distant relative who was a Sister Tutor at the local county hospital, armed with a bundle of prospectuses from the different London hospitals, and was told to pick the one with the uniform she liked the best and apply. She remembers that the pamphlets were quite glossy and all featured pictures of nurses in heeled shoes. Her mother's female relatives, many of whom had spent their lives in service as ladies' maids and nannies in various big houses, approved of her choice of career but, like her father, only because she had been accepted by a London teaching hospital.

Most women who remembered an early image of nursing associated it with their own experiences of sickness, relatives' experiences of sickness, or female relatives who worked as nurses in one form or another. These memories emphasise the more practical dimensions of women's lived experiences, and dismiss notions of romantic vocationalism instilled by popular images and stories. Ly was influenced by her godmother who was a midwife, V by friends who were nurses, M by caring for an elderly relative; MS's mother was a Sister with ambitions for her daughter's future. Only two people claimed they had always wanted to be nurses; only one thought that she had been born to it, that nursing was 'innate'. Nursing was initially seen as a job by most of the interviewees, rather than as a career. Of the two women who claimed that they had always wanted to be nurses, one of them thought that this was due to a lack of alternative role models. For some, nursing was a preferable option to working in a factory or an office or a bank. Those who had a clear image of what it would be like to be a nurse had personally experienced nursing care, or had nursed relatives or knew relatives or friends who were nurses. Only two people remembered seeing any recruitment literature; only one person remembered reading a nursing career novel. Other popular images, such as films, early television programmes, medical romances and magazine stories seemed to have had little impact on the memories of any of the interviewees.

Drumming it into you: the battleaxes

In a detailed participant observation study of professional assimilation, Kath Melia calls attention to the way that the student nurses she studied consciously 'fitted in' to the ward environment in order to get by (Melia 1987). The following accounts reveal a similar strategy, with trainees attempting to 'fit in' to a militaristic, matriarchal structure that was common throughout the hospital nursing system at the time in spite of historical differences at the institutional level. Although there were variations in the training programmes on offer, a quasi-military structure of discipline permeated the organisation of nurse training. This was maintained by a system where ward Sisters had a reasonable degree of autonomy, and often remained in post for most of their working lives. Images of nurses as either the handmaidens of doctors or self-sacrificing angels are most inappropriate when applied to this group. The two images that stand out in relation to the Sisters are bossy but kindly motherly figures and punitive authoritarian spinsters. Nightingale's rhetorical concepts materialise as flesh and blood characters in the 'battleaxe' Sisters, an image that cropped up repeatedly in all of the interviews.

The 'battleaxe' is typically a middle-aged spinster who has worked as a Sister on the same ward for many years, and runs it with the efficiency of a military campaign:

'I was very, very young and very naive ... and there was this battleaxe of a ward Sister who ran the ward like a military operation' (J).

'The Sisters would put the fear of God into you ... the old regimental ones used to put the fear of God into you' (Ly).

'She [the Sister] always liked to be shouting at you ... she's more or less like a sergeant major, yeh?' (V).

Or she might be the Sister Tutor, in charge of the trainee nurses:

'If the Sister Tutor was coming you would, you know, stand at attention and all this. Sister Tutor was real cruel looking, she was strict looking and we were scared of her' (G).

Sometimes, a younger Sister fitted the stereotype:

'Some of the Sisters mortified some of the nurses ... there was no need to make them feel like that. I hated the Sister on Clitheroe Ward, I think everybody did. She was young but she was cruel. I thought how can you be so cruel, we were so frightened' (O).

Although 'battleaxes' could be frightening, they are also remembered for their clarity of judgement, their kindness and their professional skills:

'Most of the best ones were battleaxes, they were really good, cared for their patients, nobody was ever overlooked or neglected. They had always worked there, you made your career out of being a ward Sister didn't you. With the ones who ran their regimes you knew exactly where you were' (J).

'She was the ward Sister when I first went there, a very fierce sort of person but very kindly; the balance was there and you felt very safe with her' (SC).

This feeling of safety was clearly a vital one in terms of giving trainee nurses the confidence to be able to carry out their work. 'Battleaxes' who were well organised, ran their wards calmly and efficiently and were kind to the patients are on the whole remembered fondly; on the other hand,

'There were some really awful people, it seemed no matter what you did you couldn't win, very sadistic' (SC).

The image of the 'battleaxe' is a potent one. The ward Sisters and Sister Tutors were role models for young trainees; as J comments,

'It wasn't that I was impressed with them, but it was persuasive, you couldn't ignore these people.'

SC thinks that the training approach was basically paternalistic, in that the Sisters not only looked after their charges but tried to model them to fit their own ideals.

The hierarchical relationships and the enforced discipline of hospital life left some nurses feeling disaffected. Instead of feeling empowered by the training process, they felt undermined by it:

'People were constantly knocking you down all the time ... they seemed to want to discourage any feelings of individual strength ... the hierarchy was very much in evidence, and you were seen to be low down ... the attitude seemed to be that we had to do this and get on with it, we had it hard, so you'll have it hard too. I got that feeling a lot during my training' (Ju).

In some cases, this 'toughening up' process had the opposite effects to those intended. Some trainees, like Dickens, abandoned their training and left nursing. Others vowed they would be different, and make changes for the better:

> 'I honestly thought when I get to the top I shall be kinder, I would never want to put anybody through what I went through, never' (O).

The interviewees' strongest collective memory was undoubtedly that of the battleaxe; these nurses were both respected and feared, fondly remembered as well as mocked. At best, they could be supportive and reassuring, at worst they could cruelly demolish a young trainee nurse's fragile sense of self.

'Battleaxes' are potent images in popular fictions, ranging from comedic figures such as Hattie Jacques in *Carry On Matron* to sadistic figures like Nurse Rachet in *One Flew Over the Cuckoo's Nest*. Few of the images are complimentary; career nurses, on the whole, were not kindly constructed throughout this period, perhaps because of more general trends to discredit career women in the public imaginary (Haskell 1974, Wilson 1980). Nurses themselves are more ambivalent about their relationship with authority figures; what seems to have provoked the most discontent is not so much being subjected to discipline, but being made to feel an inferior and incompetent member of a rigid hierarchy. As one interviewee put it, 'they seemed to want to discourage any feelings of individual strength' (Ju). Most of the interviewees felt that they were actively deterred from questioning things, from using their initiative; 'it was drilled out of us' (Ju).

In her autobiography, Markham (1975) describes how every aspect of hospital life was deeply permeated by this sense of hierarchy. Speaking to the medical staff, let alone fraternising with them, was completely out of the question for anyone below the rank of Sister, and she dismisses doctor/nurse romance novels as pure fiction. Trainee and auxiliary nurses claim similar experiences of subservience – to doctors, other nursing staff, para-medical staff and domestic staff.

> 'If you were a greybelt [first year] you were actually not only bottom of the nursing pile but at the bottom of every other pile that was going as well' (J).

> 'You were treated just like you didn't exist, left with all the mess to clear up, never thanked, never asked, always told . . .' (Ju).

The romanticised 'handmaiden' image of nursing is one that these interviewees reacted strongly against. No-one denied that the image existed, only that:

'Nurse and doctor story books painted a completely different image
. . . I suppose they could make it up to seem ever so romantic and
nice . . . it is not that way in reality' (M).

SC felt that 'it was a load of old rubbish, it made me decide not to marry
a doctor very early on, they were the biggest rogues'.

Markham describes the rigours of nursing life at this time; the lack of
disposable goods and equipment now taken for granted, such as inconti-
nence pads, tissues and cotton wool, made the work dirtier, more menial,
and more arduous. Her graphic accounts of clearing up faeces and other
human emissions and the descriptions of her reactions to this 'dirty' work
fill a gap in nursing's official histories. After describing in some detail the
emptying and cleaning of the sputum mugs, she comments, 'Even now, I
clench my teeth and keep a firm grip on my stomach when I recall that
"plop" as they emptied' (1975: 149).

Many of the interviewees undertaking general training felt that in some
ways they were badly abused, asked to take on far too much responsibility
before they had sufficient experience and training; 'the feeling of being
responsible really was a lot, I think it was too much too early' (Ju). In
addition, all trainees had to do their share of the dirty work; 'We were
treated like skivvies, it was easier to give the job to me, I had to do a lot
of unpleasant things' (MS). Ly recalls that she was frightened about a
number of things during training but 'there wasn't much support for nurses
at all, people were very hard and cold . . .'. Coping alone on the ward on
night duty, or with just one other junior nurse, was a common experience;
'night duty was always quite stressful . . . we were put in charge of a ward
quite early [in our training] because of staff shortages' (Ju). 'We didn't
realise what kind of responsibility we were taking on and we'd just do it'
(Ly).

These feelings were closely connected with fears about facing death, and
coping with the bodies of others. Individuals had different reactions to the
practicalities of nursing work that ranged from dealing with personal feelings of disgust (that the work was in some way beneath them) to coping
with the paraphernalia of surgical and medical intervention (drains, drips,
irrigations, suction and so on). Ju sums up these feelings succinctly:

'I remember being terrified a lot of times when I was training.
Even doing a bed bath at the beginning was quite scary, I mean
you're eighteen years old and you haven't dealt with other people's
bodies . . . and they're depending on you in a way that is completely
new to you.'

In spite of their criticisms of undergoing training in the 'old school',
most of the interviewees had reservations about recent modernisations.

Although authoritarian hierarchies pervaded early nursing life without exception, suffusing both public duty on the wards and private life in the nursing home, the rule-bound framework created a feeling of security, particularly for someone arriving in England from elsewhere.

> 'It was very secure and protective really, we didn't even need to go outside the hospital; they looked after the nurses very well, better than what we do today' (O).

At the age of 17, SC was made a ward of Matron when her parents emigrated to Canada:

> 'As a cadet nurse we were protected if you like so that they could keep an eye on these tender young girls. I suppose it was a paternalistic approach, I mean if they looked after us, we came up with the goods.'

The closed and regulated life did have some compensations, primarily the enduring friendships that developed out of a sense of shared adversity and common fears amongst those in your 'set'. A 'set' was a cohort group who began their training together. The rigid hierarchy demarcated the various stages of training each 'set' had reached by various symbols of increased authority, usually in the form of stripes, belts or dress colour. Fraternisation between different 'sets' was actively discouraged; as a result, the group formed strong friendship bonds that acted as a support network:

> 'When you went off duty, everybody was in the same boat, we always knew there was somebody there ...' (O).

> 'I had a very close group of friends, people tended to cluster in groups ... there wasn't much mixing outside of one's own group. Out of the forty-six that started, there's still thirty-six of us that keep in contact regularly and we meet up every other year. We were a terribly cohesive group' (J).

> 'We made friends then, and we're still friends now. What I'd do without my best mate, I don't know' (SA).

On the other hand, the long hours of work and shift systems tended to militate against a healthy social life, creating an insular lifestyle. Living and working with nurses tended, as Dickens noted, not to make people very outgoing or independent; it was a tight knit, closed community. MS sums up a general feeling amongst all the interviewees when she comments,

'I wouldn't have survived without my peers . . . we were kind to each other weren't we.'

All the interviewees have remained in contact with at least one or two people that they trained with, a testimony to the strength of the friendship bonds forged between those who shared the demanding experience of becoming nurses.

Out of place: re-location, racism and the 'other'

The experiences of those who came to Britain to train and work as nurses in the 1950s and 1960s are deeply hidden in the margins of other narratives, other discourses. The earliest image of a black nurse in a British film is in *Sapphire* (GB 1959), a 'social problem' film that attempts to tackle racist issues; the nurse has a tiny, walk-on role and a middle-class English accent. In the doctor/nurse romance literature, the earliest image I found is in Bess Norton's *Night Duty at Dukes* (1960). Here the black nurse Theo is given a thoroughly white middle-class identity, emphasised by her ambition to marry a white middle-class man. It is not until the televising of *Angels* in the mid-1970s that black nurses begin to feature more prominently as characters in fictional dramas, although in Peter Nicols' bitingly satirical film *The National Health or Nurse Norton's Affair* (1973) a black nurse is one of the central characters. There are no published autobiographical works written by black nurses working in post-war Britain, although researchers Bryan, Dadzie and Scafe (1985) have recorded and compiled an oral history of black women's lives in Britain which features two accounts by nurses. Torkington (1985) and Baxter (1988) have counteracted institutionally racist accounts of black women's experiences in the health services through researching personal narratives of their working lives. These works re-locate black women as the subjects of their own discourse, rather than as the objects of white speculation and interpretation. The loss of specificity across a range of representations and discourses continues to deny black nurses voices of their own and a secure place in nursing history in spite of their large numbers in the workforce; for the most part the problems faced by black nurses are unevenly tackled by employers and professional organisations (Beishon, Virdee and Hagell 1995). In contrast, white male nurses (a much smaller group) are officially recognised as a minority within nursing in need of special career incentives and support.[18]

On the odd occasion when the presence of black nursing staff has been officially recognised, it has tended to situate 'them' as 'problems', people who could not 'fit in' to the hospital system. In her review of the literature on recruitment and attrition, MacGuire found only one study that researched black nurses' experiences of their training. The researcher concluded that cultural differences were the primary cause of disaffiliation by black nurses, that they had difficulty in assimilating hospital routine as well as adjusting to life in Britain more generally (Martin 1965). As Ly commented in conversation after her interview, the main problem that black nurses have had to face in England is being seen differently, being seen as outsiders. One of the problems this group has is that until recently both public and professional images of black nursing identity in Britain were very marginalised and, as a result, not available as role models to young people. Arriving in Britain, trainees were confronted with white images of nursing which projected the same discourse of nursing values to that promoted, for example, in Barbados, but whereas the latter had been the focus of aspiration, the white image was disorientating. The nurses' uniform was a symbol of personal achievement and status, but it provided scant protection from constant racial harassment. Ly's memory of the image of her godmother has helped to keep alive her belief in her innate ability to nurse, against the problems of struggling to achieve her ambitions in institutions dominated by ideologies of whiteness.[19]

In *Behind the Screens*, Jocelyn Lawler discusses at some length how female nurses manage the problem of unbridled male sexuality when they are intimately caring for male patients. Lawler considers that male patients sometimes act in this way because 'sexuality is a pervasive aspect of social life and almost any situation is a potential occasion for sexual expression' (Lawler 1991: 213). Arguably, in British society, racism is also a pervasive aspect of social life, and almost any occasion can provide the potential for the expression of racial prejudice and hatred. Black nurses have to manage situations at work where both patients and colleagues of either sex react in relation to their 'blackness'. In this respect, all the nurses interviewed here found 'managing' their white nursing peers and hospital management teams far more difficult than managing racist reactions from their patients.

Other sections of this chapter bury the specificity of black experiences within general accounts of the image of the ministering angel, the battleaxe and the sexy nurse. These images present problems for black nurses that are not immediately obvious; for example, the image of the battleaxe was a recurring one in their accounts, as it was for most of the white nurses, but whereas for white nurses the battleaxe represents a history of class-based military authority, for black nurses it continues to resonate with an image of white oppression and colonial rule. Several of the interviewees point out the absence of black nurses in positions of power and responsibility in English hospitals compared with their concentration in the lower grades of the least prestigious areas of nursing, such as geriatrics and psychiatric care. As I pointed out in Chapter 3, where the prestige attached to cure is low and care is viewed as a curatorial or custodial activity, nursing has traditionally tended to be organised on a task-centred basis that isolates the most physically demanding and the dirtiest jobs. This hierarchical care structure reinforces notions about the low status of geriatric nursing in the profession, a status that is reflected in the salary scales and 'glass ceilings' on professional progress. The nurses interviewed here point out how their ethnicity and gender has trapped them in the lower staffing grades in the lowest status areas of the nursing profession.

The historian Carolyn Steedman claims that: 'Personal interpretations of past time – the stories people tell themselves in order to explain how they got to the place they currently inhabit – are often in deep and ambiguous conflict with the official interpretative devices of a culture' (Steedman 1986: 6). This is particularly true of the stories told by this group; their systems of beliefs and values are deeply immersed in the official discourses and ideologies of professional nursing but they nonetheless find themselves excluded from that discourse and denied a voice or a place from which they can speak. The accounts that follow were told to me by four women who came from Barbados to train as nurses in English hospitals between the early 1950s and the late 1960s. Their desire to tell their stories was strong, even though there was an awareness (and a degree of scepticism) about how their accounts would inevitably be mediated through the official interpretative device of my white standpoint.[20] The stories have been told on the understanding that one day they might contribute to a history of black nurses' lives in Britain written by a black nursing scholar.

In the synopsis which follows, the mediating frameworks I have used in order to present the interviews are important interpretative considerations. I decided before I began the interviewing process that I would use the same questions for all the participants as a basic framework for discussion and that I would avoid asking 'leading' questions, particularly on issues of difference. In theory, I thought this would leave individuals free to steer a course through the interview without feeling too directed by my assessment of what the important issues were. In practice, two interviewees made it clear to me before we began to talk that they wanted to discuss racial issues in nursing.

The problems inherent in any transcription process from oral to written form are compounded if the interviewer and interviewee do not share a common cultural background. This is a particularly important issue, given that 'otherness' to nursing's white middle-class ideal has invariably been presented in fictional texts through the use of different speech idioms in the form of heavy accents and dialects. In the *Sue Barton* books, for example, accent is used as a metonym for outsider status in society; the 'waif' Marianne whom Sue 'saves' from a life on the streets of New York is represented as heavily accented in the initial stories, but as she gradually assimilates a white identity, her guttural accent disappears. In *Night Duty at Dukes* assimilation into nursing's white middle-class ideal denies Theo, who is from Jamaica, any pleasure or pride in her own cultural identity. Although nobody amongst the interview group singled out accent and dialect as a specific problem, it is an important aspect of the differential power relations inscribed in the processes of mediation and interpretation.[21]

What follows is my understanding of the stories which, for reasons of clarity of analysis and presentation, are summarised and divided into three sections which outline various stages of engagement with nursing images, ideals and practices. The interviewees throw some light on to the question of what happens to self-image when dominant discourses do not correspond to lived experience, when the gap between self-perception of one's own professional identity and the public and professional image of that self grows ever more unbridgeable. The sense of outrage felt by the interviewees is not directed at nursing's idealised conception of itself, but at the organisation of nursing practice and its complicity with the institutional racism embedded in the NHS. The latter in particular is viewed as the villain of the piece for refusing to tackle the racist ideologies inherent within its system of institutional care.[22]

Early images

Early images of nursing tend to have come from female friends and relatives at home in Barbados, some of whom were nurses themselves, some of whom wanted their daughters to be nurses. Playing games pretending to be nurses and doctors was quite popular. Three people had wanted to be nurses from when they were quite young. Ly was most influenced by her godmother who was a midwife:

> 'She was a very bubbly and loving type of person so she would always come around and see you from time to time and I would see her walk in with this crisp white apron and a little like straw basket over her arm and just go round the village visiting people.'

Some people had vague memories of reading books about nursing, but thought that they had not been at all influenced by popular stories and magazines. One person remembered reading doctor/nurse romances, which 'painted a completely different image in the book than what in reality it is' (M).

Amongst this very small group, there seems to be little apparent difference to me between their early images, hopes and aspirations and those of some of the white interviewees. In Barbados nursing was viewed as a relatively high status occupation for women; the image of nursing seems to have had a great deal in common with that projected by the London teaching hospitals, promoting personal qualities of patience, self-sacrifice and service to a higher ideal. It was a difficult profession to enter with limited opportunities for training:

'The nurses there ... they were proud. They were proud girls to be nurses. Anybody who got into the nursing profession there were more or less respected and they were proud' (M).

When opportunities opened up for training in Britain, for some it seemed to offer a chance of realising aspirations which might otherwise have remained unfulfilled at home. To train as a nurse in Barbados, you needed to come from quite a wealthy family; for young upwardly aspirant Barbadian women, the opportunity of training as a nurse in Britain seemed an ideal way to achieve a coveted ambition.

Recruitment and training

There is no doubt that these personal aspirations were embers of ambition fanned by recruiters to persuade young women to leave their homes and train in Britain, although the actual mechanisms of the recruitment process are only partially revealed in the accounts below. People came to nurse in Britain through a range of different routes. V was given a copy of a British nursing journal, the *Nursing Mirror*, by a friend; she wrote and applied to three hospitals in the south of England, all of whom accepted her. Rather than going through the formalities of government sponsorship, her parents paid her travelling costs. G and her friends responded to a government-led recruitment drive. She remembers hearing about it on the radio, and through the careers service at school. Ly arrived in England to join her mother, a nursing auxiliary, when she was almost 15. She decided that she would become a nurse, and applied for training at a local hospital as soon as she was 16. M came to England to join her boyfriend, writing to several hospitals in the hope of starting her training, but she was un- successful. She married, had her children and began working as a nursing auxiliary in the early 1970s.

Many people seem to have been unaware that there were two forms of nurse training available in Britain. In Barbados, only training for state regis- tration (general nursing) was available, and only state registered nurses were employed, therefore becoming an enrolled nurse was not useful for anyone wanting to return home. G claims that decisions about who did what training were made in a fairly arbitrary way by Barbadian government employees:

'A lot of us didn't know until we got here. They never let us know over there. And they used to decide – favouritism I guess – who they sent to do enrolled nursing and who they sent to do the General' (G).

G claims that a lot of people ended up in her situation, spending two years training for the roll, who had sufficient educational qualifications for general training. Because she was on contract to the hospital, she had no option other than to complete the two years and get her certificate before she could start her general training; 'I was determined that as soon as I finished, I was going to do my general.' Enrolled nurses had to go back on student pay whilst general training, and were only allowed six months off the three-year training period for their existing qualifications. This was an added disincentive to take up training for nurses like V who had to support their families, whether they were living in Britain or, as was sometimes the case, at home in Barbados:

> 'After a few months I was thinking about doing my training but the pay you got was so small I couldn't afford to do my training then . . . the wages at the end of the month are only eight or nine pounds . . .'

V shared a room with two other women in a similar situation to herself who had to send money home for the care of their children and, in conse-quence, could not afford to give up their auxiliary nursing jobs to train.

Some people commented on the fear and strangeness they felt when they arrived in Britain. G remembers how she didn't like England when she arrived in 1961, and how strange she felt 'because everybody was white'. In conversation after the interview, V told me that she felt as if she was going to be eaten alive by white people when she got off the boat, but that going to the hospital offered a sense of some security. Both V and G started work almost immediately after their arrival at the hospital, only a day or two after they had arrived in England. Although she was wearing the coveted nurse's uniform V initially found the work distasteful; she had not expected to be dealing with so many elderly, incontinent people. G found herself in a small country hospital working with eight other black nurses; looking back now, she thinks she was lucky going to Yorkshire because people were very friendly.

One of the significant differences between the training experiences of black and white nurses lies in their social lives. The white nurses recalled how their social lives had revolved around their own cohort groups, and that they rarely mixed with those outside their own set. The positive side of this was the strong bonds forged between women which have been carried into their later lives. Black nurses tended to ignore the peer group hierarchy, bonding across sets and national boundaries to form networks of support:

> 'I felt strange but it was nice because . . . there was eight other black girls there. As soon as they heard the new ones were in they came to introduce themselves. And they were around to let us feel at home. But we were very homesick' (G).

Ly remembers having a healthy social life:

> 'There were girls from Jamaica, Trinidad, Bermuda, and there were lots of colleagues from Mauritius and lots from the Caribbean Islands so it was quite interesting.'

In addition, there were staff in the hospital kitchens from Greece, Spain and Italy. V remembers a good atmosphere, taking turns in off-duty time to cook food to share with the others, courtesy of a local butcher who used to provide cheap meat for the nursing staff.

Experiences of training were in some ways similar to those of white nurses; people recounted similar stories about their place in nursing's hierarchy, with authoritarian Sisters and autocratic medical staff figuring in similar ways. V remembers learning many of her basic nursing skills from one Sister in particular, who made no distinction between what she taught to auxiliaries and pupil nurses. G, at a hospital in Yorkshire in the early 1960s, found the people warm and friendly even though the Sisters were daunting. V remembers one Sister who always picked on black nurses, 'she always liked to be shouting at you', but otherwise remembers being treated with respect. M found herself working with a nursing officer who always found fault with the black nurses, rarely with the white:

> 'I know I'm an auxiliary, I know I'm lower down the scale, but she made me feel so ... oh ... she wasn't nice at all.'

Working with somebody who was determined to find fault was clearly an undermining experience during the early days of training/working, but for this group of women it was the nurses' re-grading exercise in the mid-1980s that finally undermined them after many years of coping with day-to-day racial harassment. (In the wake of the Griffith Report, posts in nursing management were abolished and nurses' posts re-graded according to the levels of responsibility they carried. Many nurses felt that the re-gradings did not adequately reflect the responsibility they exercised in their work, resulting in bitter battles with the employers. For a detailed account see Buchan *et al.* 1989.)

Reflections on a life in nursing

Overseas students had to cope not only with the disappointments of arriving in Britain and finding it a very different place from the idealised conceptions of the 'mother country' they had been taught to expect at school, but also with working in a system of health care that fell well below their expectations. M pointed out how the British system of caring for the elderly in old-fashioned and poorly equipped geriatric hospitals seemed quite uncivilised compared with Barbadian standards:

'It was shocking at the beginning. They thought that we – West Indians – were primitive, but when I came to the hospital it was more primitive than what we had ...'

M recalls that at that time,

'nobody wanted to work in geriatrics, nobody. I think they wanted people coming to England to work on geriatrics.'

M worked with two SENs caring for fifty-two elderly people on two wards while they taught her basic nursing care; she remained in geriatric nursing for eighteen years. A particular milestone for the large black workforce in geriatric nursing was the move for unionisation in 1974/5:

'We had a coloured bloke who came working at the hospital, and he was a charge nurse and he started up the union. Well, there might have been a union before, but nobody came to us ... And it was only when the union came along that the staff begin to increase ...' (M).

Like the other women interviewed here, M has steered her daughter away from a career in nursing; she feels that the changes in the NHS are making things worse for nurses, who are being asked to work more hours for the same pay.

'They haven't said anything about redundancy yet, but what has come up now, they given us part-timers – I work thirty hours a week – this is what I understand it to be, that every nineteen weeks we work one night without pay.'

The sense of outrage felt by M at the low value placed on her years of hard work and commitment to the NHS is echoed by the other interviewees. Ly now works as a staff nurse on a surgical ward after sixteen years on night duty in a special care baby unit. Commenting on the fact that overseas nurses were placed mainly on the geriatric wards, Ly felt that the price paid for this was that they gained only limited experience of medical and surgical nursing which made it difficult for them to move. Ly sees the nurses' re-grading exercise in the mid-1980s as something of a victory for those working in this traditionally undervalued area of nursing because SENs were finally given recognition for running wards and being responsible for large numbers of elderly ill patients. Apart from this small victory for the large black workforce, she thinks it is very hard for a black nurse to move up the career ladder; white nurses dominate nursing management out of all proportion to their numbers overall:

'I think really that black nurses realised that this was happening and that they weren't getting anywhere fast and they opted out. I notice that there aren't as many in nursing.'

Ly is deeply frustrated that in spite of achieving state registration and taking extra courses, she has been unable to fulfil her aspirations in nursing:

'I'm the last person to have a chip on my shoulder, but it does seem that once you're black it's ten times harder to move.'

She thinks that nursing is less attractive as a career for women these days unless they want to move into management or specialise in an off-shoot area like health promotion. Her 12-year-old daughter has ambitions to be a lawyer.

V has spent most of her working life as an auxiliary nurse and is now looking forward to retirement. In spite of many years of experience of caring for elderly patients, she has to carry out the instructions of student nurses who are still at college and have very little experience on the wards. Her knowledge and skills are ignored, making her feel undervalued and regretful that she didn't do her training:

'You get some young little staff that just come out [of college], maybe I was a nurse before they were born, and, oh, want to push you around, and it makes me feel sad.'

V thinks that they're 'trying to do nursing by paper' and that nurses no longer provide the levels of physical care that they used to, even though there are more staff on the wards.

'Sometimes you go to the ward, you can't get a cake of soap, there's no dettol, there's no savlon . . . it's awful. Now the patients can't even get a slice of bread. There's no breakfast coming out, no bacon or eggs and I think it is wrong for the old people because they have worked all of their years and at the end of their life, they should get treated better . . .'

G worked as a Sister on a gynaecological ward for twelve years, and is now having a rest from the NHS, which she thinks has become a deeply racist institution. Although she agrees that the nurses' re-grading exercise did benefit some black nurses, it was also used to discriminate against them. G was the senior Sister on her ward by many years, but she was given a lower grading (and hence a lower salary) than her white co-worker. Her tribunal appeal was never heard. As the cuts in health services started to be severely felt at ward level, morale amongst the nursing staff fell and tensions between the staff grew. G decided to take early retirement while she was still young enough to get another job. She can provide numerous examples of the poor treatment black nursing staff received during re-grading at her hospital and the preferential treatment shown to whites.

G is highly critical of government policy and the effects that the new internal market in health care services is having at the level of day-to-day management of patient care:

> 'Patients were complaining that their food was shocking, and the wards weren't clean because they'd cut back on cleaning and domestic staff . . . they expected one person to do the work that three people used to do. Impossible.'

Her views on the changes in the education and training of nurses are similar to those of others in this study; that college and degree-level trainings do not equip nurses properly with the skills they need to be able to do their job. Like the other women here, she would not be keen for her daughter to take up nursing in the health service. This short study therefore entirely supports Baxter's thesis that the black nurse is an endangered species unless the health service can prove to those who remain that it values the contri-bution of black nurses.[23] The opinion of these nurses is that to date this has not been shown to be the case.

The problems of subsuming the experiences of all female nurses under a generalist rubric are clear. The social histories of nursing need to include the contributions that black nurses have made to the profession, and the diffi-culties that they have had to overcome. As a profession that has been shaped by discourses of class and gender rather than the possession of a particular, specialist body of scientific knowledge, professional nursing has always been torn between striving for status through education and training, and trying to achieve it by proving managerial ability through control of the (largely) female workforce who do nursing work. Both of these projects involve one group of people subjugating an 'other'. Achieving recognition in the pro-fession has tended to mean specialising in either education or management, leaving those who wished to develop their practical expertise in caring skills without a clear career path once they obtained their registration. This struc-ture was a particularly invidious one for those arriving to train as nurses from Britain's former colonies. Not only did they end up working in the least prestigious areas of the health service which have always been notoriously under-funded and under-staffed, but once there, they were caught in a financial trap. For some black nurses, their ambitions to enter the profession as registered nurses ended, cruelly squashed by a combination of low pay, low status and long hours of hard and dirty work.

In an analysis of the racial division of reproductive labour in the United States, Evelyn Nakano Glenn points out that 'race' has tended to be analysed in academic feminism as an additional oppression to that of class, rather than as an integrated element of class and gender exploitation. Glenn argues that in the first half of the twentieth century, racial-ethnic women were employed as servants in white households to relieve middle-class women of the more onerous aspects of reproductive labour. With the expansion of the commodified service sector in the second half of the century, racial-ethnic women were disproportionately employed in lower level service work, whilst white women filled the cleaner, white collar supervisory and lower professional positions. The division of labour in the household is mirrored by the division of labour in the public sphere, where racial-ethnic women are employed to do the unseen and heavy, dirty servicing work such as cooking, cleaning and caring for the elderly and the chronic sick. Glenn argues that with the shift of domestic labour from the private to the public sphere, a face-to-face hierarchy has been replaced by a structural hierarchy. She illustrates her points using a study of stratification in the nursing labour force, pointing out how white RNs (the equivalent of registered general nurses in Britain) are over-represented in the top grades in relation to nursing numbers overall, whilst racial-ethnic women are disproportionately represented in the lower grades of nurses' aid (the equivalent of an auxiliary).

In Britain, as Stones (1972) has pointed out, black male and female nurses were often employed in low status specialist areas such as psychiatry where male nurses were traditionally employed. In terms of K. Williams' (1978) model, black nurses were placed in positions of custodial care, with the underlying implication that black female nurses were not only 'closer to nature' than their white counterparts, but also masculinised. The barriers to their progress, although ostensibly presented as educational and cultural, were essentially ideological: nursing's professional ideal of white middle-class femininity. The NHS increasingly relied on the low paid labour of black women (and some men) to sustain and maintain a system that promised care to white Britons from 'the cradle to the grave'. To meet the provisions of this social contract, black labour was imported from the former British 'colonies' under the auspices of 'training' and 'aid'. Many of those who came to Britain believed that they would be able to train as nurses, and return home. Instead, they found themselves trapped by contracts, low wages, and non-viable qualifications with no means of redress. In this way, they continued to be subservient to the power that had colonised them, doing the dirty work on which a more 'caring' (white) society was being built.[24]

Institutional structures buffer and mediate the relationship between those who do the dirty work and those who benefit from that work. The institutional care of, for example, elderly white people by black nurses clearly benefits white women, who would otherwise have to shoulder this burden of reproductive labour. In Britain, this burden was traditionally carried by

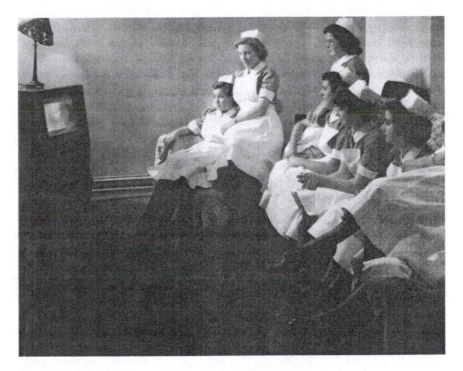

Figure 4.2 Nurses' Home, Liverpool, late 1950s

women from the lower social classes and Irish immigrant labour who formed the bulk of the nursing staff in the former workhouses and municipal hospitals. When there was insufficient local labour to staff these institutions, nursing managers 'sent for a boatload from Barbados' (Rose, personal communication 1992) to make good the shortfall. As White (1985b) has pointed out, successful management was judged in terms of ensuring there was a constant supply of labour to meet the demands of care. In this institutional hierarchy, class, gender and race became an intertwining nexus of structural determinants that shaped the lives and careers of black women in British nursing.

The 'proper' nurse: self as image, image as self

> For those who survive the basic training course, personal identity is inextricably bound up with identity as a nurse.
>
> (MacGuire 1969: 107)

Two further concerns are central to understanding the self-image of female nurses at this time: the first of these is an individual's mental image of the 'ideal nurse', what she considers a 'proper' nurse is or should be; the second is the relationship of these personal images to the official discourses that have constructed them. Interpretations are situated in the context of the present; accounts of past time are refracted through the relationship of the 'ideal' image to a personalised, professional sense of self existing in the present day. One way of thinking about this self is as a personal 'ideal' or image split by the critical lens of everyday nursing practice into a self constructed through officially prescribed professional ideologies and institutional determinations.

The 'proper' nurse

The concept of the 'proper' nurse is an important one in the context of a feminist analysis of images of femininity. The 'proper' nurse is a discursive formation formed and shaped by the processes of becoming and being a nurse. It is inextricably part of each individual's self-perception, the underlying framework of beliefs and attitudes that has shaped response to the interview questions. Conceptions of the 'proper' nurse are formed from a mixture of pre-nursing histories (social background, education and early working lives as schoolgirls, hairdressers, factory, shop and office workers, bank clerks and nursing cadets), experiences of training (in a range of institutions) and current working lives (as nurses and teachers, researchers, managers, midwives, psychologists and counsellors). Underlying the memories recounted to me of their earliest images of nursing, each interviewee has an image of what constitutes their idealised conception of the 'proper' nurse, an amalgam of the principal attributes that every nurse believes to be an integral aspect of her nursing self. Foundational concepts of the 'proper' nurse are initially formed during the training process; most trainees were subjected to an intensive ethical training that constantly proclaimed service to the patient as nursing's highest ideal. The split identified by White (1986) between the different discourses of professionalisers and managers is not apparent at the level of training because training was the one area of nursing securely controlled by the professionalisers.

Amongst the interviewees, it is perhaps unsurprising that those who articulated the most vivid images of a 'proper' nurse were trained at London teaching hospitals. As one interviewee commented, 'If I meet ex-London nurses I can spot a Guys' nurse anywhere, she has this arrogance' (J). Likewise, in provincial teaching hospitals, the nurses had a tendency to view themselves as superior, 'a different calibre to everyone else' (MS). Many of the teaching hospitals promoted an ethos of superiority amongst their nursing staffs based on their religious legacies of dedication, duty and devoted service and modern reputations for medical excellence. This heritage was protected and promoted by Schools of Nursing enforcing strict discipline and a programme of moral education; some nurses still had to sign a contract of moral conduct, promising not to bring the name of their hospital into disrepute, as recently as the mid-1970s. All contact with members of the opposite sex was open to scrutiny by nursing management; MS remembers being called to account by a senior nursing officer for holding a dying male patient's hand because it was deemed 'unseemly'. Other interviewees commented on the restrictions that denied all men (even fathers) access to nurses' homes:

'You had to sign in and out, you couldn't be out after a certain time without them knowing where and what time you were coming in. It was so strict it was unbearable' (Ju).

In addition to policing the living and working environments of their trainee nurses, some institutions attempted to control their off-duty time as well. Fraternising with the medical staff in off-duty hours could earn a student a sharp rebuff from a senior. Marriage was often seen as a form of betrayal, of placing personal desire before public duty.[25]

Wearing the wrong kind of clothes in public could lead to professional expulsion. J remembers that:

'there was a girl in the third year who got her photograph full length in the *Daily Express* as part of an article illustrating what the modern nurse looks like and what the modern nurse has to live on. There she was in a short skirt, long boots, looking very glamorous and she was told after this that she wouldn't pass her hospital exam . . . they wouldn't allow her to work as a staff nurse at Barts.'

Respectability was integral to professional identity; on duty, make-up and jewellery were forbidden, hair had to be worn above the collar and off the face, and shoes had to be 'sensible'.

This study reflects a very strong sense of identity formed by those who trained in teaching hospitals. Whether this is due to interviewees selecting teaching hospital training because of the image these hospitals projected, or whether this ethos was absorbed during training is more difficult to determine. MS, for example, chose to train at a teaching hospital because she wanted to overcome her feelings of inferiority as a middle-class girl in a working-class occupation (hairdressing), whereas J claims she would never have become a nurse at all if she hadn't been accepted by one of the London hospitals of her choice. Social status rather than the pursuit of educational excellence was the major factor in both their choices, underlining what one interviewee called 'the snobbishness' of these institutions.

This study can give no indication of the degree to which any particular image of the 'proper' nurse promoted by a training institution was internalised by those becoming nurses, only that there was an awareness amongst most interviewees of what the hospital's image was. J thought she developed a very strong sense of identity because there was no gap between theory and practice:

> 'We did exactly what we were taught in school. I think the sense of identity was very, very forceful, you may have took it for granted at the time, but when you get a bit away from it, you realise it gave a sense of coherence too. I think we had a very strong sense of identity, the uniform, the whole thing about training in that hospital gives a very strong sense of identity, and I think a sense of identity might be quite important' (J).

Images of the 'proper' nurse amongst most of the women that I interviewed remain close to more traditional ideals of nursing excellence, debunking more modern images of the highly skilled and educated professional at ease in a high-tech medical environment. SA expressed this as follows:

> 'All this high-tech stuff to my mind isn't nursing. An awful lot [of nurses] to my mind now don't seem to be that interested in the patient.'

This portrait of the 'proper' nurse is not as traditionally vocationalist as it might at first appear; unlike the stereotypes pictured in popular and professional discourses, the personal image is a much more complex, composite and multi-layered one. Each person's early impressions of nurses and nursing have been constantly revised and renewed in the light of experience. This means that the mental concept contains fragments of popular and professional discourses, but these are wrought by the experiences of becoming and being a nurse. SA graphically illustrates this point when she tries to describe an incident that left a lasting impression on her:

> 'I remember sitting by his bed and fighting death between us and that's what it felt like.'

This was quickly followed by,

> 'Absolutely crackers – but that's what it felt like',

to cover any embarrassment that such an intimate revelation might cause to either of us within the formality of the academic interview situation. A discourse of nurses' emotional work haunts SA's account of her training and her concept of a 'proper' nurse, but the persistent devaluation of this kind of work and its melodramatic mediation as 'tender loving care' leaves it veiled beneath an apologetic wimple of vocationalism. Hilary Graham (1983) has written about the gendered nature of caring as emotional labour undertaken by women; more recent research has attempted to analyse how nurses care in an attempt to give value and status to this under-valued aspect of nurses' work (P. Smith 1992). Most nurses are trained to hide their feelings and respect the privacy of others and this becomes internalised, a discursive formation that shapes the 'proper' nurse. In the interview situation, each person's mental image of the 'proper' nurse was constructed from fragments – from their own nursing histories, from popular stereotypes and professional ideals – creating a personal projection of the self as a nurse. Ju commented that the interview process had forced her to focus on her feelings about being a nurse; the narrative she created helped her to rethink her past and draw her experiences together.

This sense of an internal construct of an ideal image is found in the autobiographical writings of Markham and Ash. In their reflections, which span lengthy periods of their working lives, both present images of the kind of work that nurses do, and the satisfactions and frustrations that they experience, that could easily be tagged vocational. Their discourses are, however, quite different, and rest on very different premises. Markham harks back to a pre-war vocationalism that places character and personality at the centre of the nursing ideal. She quotes her list of ideal attributes from a 1930s training manual (*A Complete System of Nursing*, Millicent Ashdown, 1939):

> She must be active yet quiet and deft, methodical, reliable, careful, clean and neat, observant, intelligent, economical, possessed of self-control preserving gentleness, tact, sympathy and common sense; careful to respect professional etiquette, remembering what is due to those in authority, courteous in manner, careful to wear her uniform with spotless simplicity, with tidy hair, no jewellery, her general bearing that of military smartness; careful to be guarded in her behaviour towards doctors and students.
>
> (Markham 1975)

This image closely corresponds to Mrs Bedford Fenwick's conception of the nurse as a woman of sound character and disposition; personal initiative, patient advocacy and self-assertiveness form no part of Markham's picture. She believes that the better pay and conditions nurses achieved as a result of their militant campaign in 1974 ran the risk of attracting 'the wrong type' of young woman into nursing; it is the kind of work that can only be done by young women who possess particular personality and character traits. Evelyn Glenn (1992) points out how these traits were used in 1930s North America to prevent black nurses from becoming part of the white professional elite. In British nursing, as MacGuire's (1969) analysis reveals, these assumptions continued to underpin ideas about the kinds of women who were suitable for nursing, and are still operative today.[26]

In contrast, Ash places initiative, self-assertiveness and patient advocacy at the core of her nursing self. Ash is concerned with how escalating bureaucratic control and rising inefficiency in the hospital system has undermined nursing morale. As a senior nursing manager with responsibility for staffing the wards, Ash became aware that trained staff were leaving the profession in droves. A lack of investment in staff, equipment and resources but a continuing reliance on nurses' goodwill and self-sacrifice finally led her to take early retirement herself. Whereas Markham sees standards ebbing away as the fault of individual nurses who do not place their patients' needs at the top of their list of priorities, Ash has a greater awareness of the role played by government policy and institutional factors. Ash describes a system that is breaking down in spite of the efforts of over-worked and under-resourced staff to shore it up. Most of the nurses I interviewed supported Ash's critique:

> 'the communication between the patient and the nurse is not what it used to be . . . Now the nurses have so much paper work to do before they go off duty that they don't have time to sit down and talk to the patient' (M).

Before she left her Sister's post, G recalls that

> 'Patients were complaining that their food was shocking, and the wards weren't clean because they'd cut back on the domestic and cleaning staff . . . We all had to be mentors. We all had to be assessors. All the changes, yet you were still expected to carry on just the same.'

The strength and determination of these nurses to defend their self-image of a 'proper' nurse in the face of diminishing resources and an increasingly stressful working environment can be read as an assertive defence of personal and professional nursing values rather than a passive acceptance of institutional authority. Although it is impossible to generalise from such a small sample, it is perhaps significant that the most vehement defenders of patients' rights in this study were those who nursed the elderly and chronic sick; for various reasons, these nurses found themselves disenfranchised from nursing's white middle-class ideal.

The deep ambivalence that some of the interviewees felt about their sense of a 'nursing self' became apparent in their comments on education and training and nursing as a career for women. Personal insecurities about nursing's professional identity and social status have compounded with the effects of diminishing resources to create a fractured sense of personal and professional identity. Discourses of patient-centred care are out of step with managerial demands for financial control, with acute staffing shortages, and statistical evaluation based on cure. This has led to a range of self-protective strategies, from trying to detach oneself emotionally from the work, what Ju described as 'becoming an automaton', to a complete denial of the nursing self as in J's 'I don't identify with being a nurse anymore'.

Most of the nurses that I interviewed expressed this ambivalence about their role and their work. In spite of a very different range of experiences, there was a general feeling that standards were declining, and that they were no longer able to deliver the kind of patient care that had given them job satisfaction. Day-to-day working realities and their mental concepts of the 'proper' nurse were no longer in harmony. G put it this way:

'Nursing's not the same, not in the hospitals anyway. Everything was focusing on the money',

and Ly:

'Nursing isn't very different, nursing is more or less the same but I think all the changes and influence have come from the political side.'

Most people pointed to the conflict between an ideal image of patient-centred care and the diminishing resources that could provide it. Several people commented that nurses used to be kinder and more loving towards one another and the patients than they are now. Ju put it this way:

'There aren't the resources there to do what you want to do, you're constantly battling to get enough time to do even the basics, and it's a losing battle. You either decide that you get out or just switch off.'[27]

All the nurses I talked to had spent their working lives involved on the 'front line' of patient care before, in some cases, taking up managerial and teaching positions. Although most were critical of their own trainings, when asked about the new college-based systems of education that students now have to undertake, there was little enthusiasm for the approach. The general opinion was that although the modern nurse is more willing to question and is occasionally more assertive, she is less confident in dealing with patients, and less well equipped to deal with the toil and stress of modern hospital life. Perhaps the reason for this perception of the modern nurse is based on a generational difference of what constitutes the 'proper' nurse, since younger nurses have entered the profession informed very differently by issues of funding and finance from the previous generation.

As one interviewee ruefully commented, 'we're all expected to be care managers now'.

The 'proper' nurse constructed by the interviewees primarily centred on a caring image, one that is usually associated with 'bedside' nursing rather than a career in nursing management or education. Many commentators have pointed out that female nurses are reluctant to leave the bedside, that to no longer directly care for patients is felt to be tantamount to betraying the cause.[28] Most researchers point out that the primary cause of this apparent lack of ambition is the conflict that women face between maintaining a career and family life. For many nurses, however, a refusal to move into management or education is not just a whimsical notion that they will be 'betraying the cause', or necessarily due to conflict with family life, although these might be presented as reasons for their decisions. A refusal to manage is grounded in real fears of having to institute staffing cuts, operate disciplinary procedures and maintain morale in the face of diminishing resources and falling standards of care. As resources in hospitals have shrunk, the battle for the hearts and minds of nursing staff has been fought more bitterly between nursing management and the professionalisers, with personal concepts of what might constitute the 'proper' nurse being ripped apart in the process. While some find the reconfiguration a challenge, the nurses I talked to who were still clinical practitioners at the bedside felt disillusioned and low in morale; their work had become fragmented, its focus skewed.[29] For those who had moved up the scale to more senior positions in clinical practice, management and education, changes in the health care system have forced them to re-evaluate not only their personal conceptions of their nursing selves, but in some cases nurses' role in the health care system and the division of labour on which that role has traditionally been based.[30]

5

THE CONTEMPORARY
IMAGINATION

One of the central arguments of this book is that although the stereotypes of nursing have remained consistently within a discourse of white femininity, their meanings and implications shift over time, not least because of interventions from nurses themselves. Thus, there was a shift in the 1940s in the ethos of service away from images of vocational commitment to the profession and towards serving the nation through a commitment to the values of the emerging NHS, followed by a shift in the 1950s towards placing nursing in the service of medicine personified by nurses as handmaidens to deified doctors. Nursing's romance with medicine reached a high point in the 1960s with publishers capitalising on the demand for doctor/nurse romantic fiction and the development of medical dramas on television. Nurses were imaged as silent handmaidens and decorative sexual spectacle or satirised as authoritarian sexually frustrated spinsters. By the 1970s, nurses themselves were protesting against these images of servility and subordination, a project that gained some momentum throughout the 1980s and 1990s.

In the 1980s and 1990s this configuration was subject to a range of pressures and discursive contexts that fashioned the ways in which images of nurses and nursing could be constructed and interpreted. Changes in the structure of nurse education, a shift in health care discourse from public service to economic rationalism, and the effects of equal opportunities policies are re-shaping nursing's professional image in the context of a health service reportedly in perpetual crisis. Images of nurses circulate in a public sphere increasingly dominated by the private interests of multi-national capitalism. The public service ethos of British terrestrial television is also under pressure, responding to developments in satellite and cable services within the context of an international image market dominated by multi-national news and entertainment conglomerates.

Against this background, the discursive context that shapes my interpretation of nursing's image in the 1980s and 1990s is that of equal opportunities; equal opportunities discourse is shaped by a liberal humanist agenda that has at its core debates about the efficacy of affirmative action and positive discrimination policies and practices. How has nursing responded to the challenge of equal opportunities, given its recent history of male domination of senior posts and the virtual exclusion of black nurses from appointments in management and education? The media, and the BBC in particular, have also had to acknowledge demands for equal opportunities at the level of staffing, casting and programme production.[1] How have these internal and external discursive contexts impacted on representations and perceptions of nursing's professional identity during the 1980s and 1990s?

The condition of the NHS has generated a public discourse of crisis centred on issues of funding, waiting lists, hospital closures and a shortage of both staff and hospital beds. The era has seen an increase in medical litigation, on-going debates about the hours worked by junior doctors in hospitals, moral panics surrounding doctors who are HIV positive treating patients, crises in the number of intensive care beds available for sick children, the threatened closure of established institutions of excellence and the controversial issue of care in the community for the long-term sick and mentally ill. The internal market in health care, established to instigate competitive tendering within the NHS and flagged as the solution to problems of waste and inefficiency, has failed to deliver the promised improvement in services, generating fierce debate and campaigns against cuts and closures in many areas of Britain. The general ethos in the 1990s has been one of crisis, a time when the changes instigated in the 1980s have come home to roost in what was once the 'jewel in the crown' of the post-war settlement and the keystone of the British welfare state.

Recruitment in crisis

If Florence Nightingale were carrying her lamp through the corridors of the NHS today she would almost certainly be looking for the people in charge.

(Roy Griffith 1983)

The 1980s will be remembered by many in Britain as the years when Prime Minister Margaret Thatcher and her successive governments decided to dismantle the post-war settlement, rolling back the frontiers of the 'nanny' state in the interests of severing what was perceived as an over-dependency on welfare and state benefits. There was, however, greater caution in their attitude to and treatment of the NHS, in part because of its popularity amongst voters but also because of the deeply embedded intransigence of medical power. Reform of the system began slowly, gathering momentum throughout the decade, culminating in the introduction of an internal market within the NHS following the government White Paper *Working for Patients* in 1989. Nurses, the largest group of NHS employees, were inevitably involved in implementing re-organisation strategies but rather than taking an active role in policy making they were caught in the cross-fire between doctors and managers (Davies 1995). What is striking, in retrospect, is the extent to which, as in the post-war period, nurses had very little influence on the policy making process, although they did secure the reform of nurse education and re-grading of nurses' jobs.[2] A thumbnail sketch of these changes provides the background against which images of nurses are figured and interpreted throughout these years and into the early 1990s.[3]

The newly elected Conservative government of 1979 was presented with the report of a Royal Commission on the NHS only two months after it took office. Celia Davies points out that at this stage there were few indications of the radical changes that lay ahead, but a number of initiatives were introduced that aimed to limit the NHS budget. In 1982, a new performance review procedure was set in place: in 1983 asset management of NHS land and property was reviewed and audit procedures were examined to ensure a more efficient use of resources. In the autumn, all laundry, domestic and catering work, 'part and parcel of the NHS as it had been understood since 1948', were put out to competitive tender (Davies 1995: 158). The cost of escalating manpower[4] led to the government creating a management enquiry team of leading business people chaired by the Sainsbury supermarket chief Roy Griffith. Griffith advocated establishing general managers at Region, District and Unit levels to replace the multi-disciplinary consensus managerial teams. These people were to be recruited from outside the NHS as well as from within; contracts were for three years and managers subject to performance review and performance-related pay. In spite of resistance from doctors, nurses and some government departments, by the end of 1985 the general managers were in place. Some commentators (for example Butler 1993: 56, quoted in Davies 1995) see the Griffith reforms as the introduction of a strong and centralised management structure that laid the foundations for the internal market that was to follow (Davies 1995: 160–1).

The publication of the government White Paper *Working for Patients* in 1989 heralded the creation of the purchaser/provider split. District Health Authorities became responsible for commissioning and purchasing health care for local residents, organising contractual arrangements for the provision of care and specifications concerning the volume, cost and quantity of provision. A new group of purchasers were created alongside them, general practitioner fundholders, who could apply directly to the Region for their own budgets with which they could purchase hospital care for their patients. It was also possible for units, called NHS Trusts, to have self-governing status and be financially self-contained; those who did not wish for trust status remained as directly managed units competing with Trusts as service providers, along with private sector companies. Davies concludes that the events of the 1980s 'seemed to show that it was impossible to move the NHS out into the market place. The solution . . . was to bring the market to the NHS' (Davies 1995: 162). She argues cogently that the aim of the Griffith reforms was to challenge medical power; general managers were introduced to curb the costs of medical care. Nursing was unimportant, insignificant, a matter of staffing the service: nurses were shut out and the structures of nursing management 'swept clean away' (Davies 1995: 163).

Throughout her account Davies emphasises that nurses are invisible to policy makers not because nurses are necessarily women but because nursing, as a profession, is gendered female. Employed by nursing's central governing body, the United Kingdom Central Council for Nursing and Midwifery (UKCC),[5] Davies was closely involved in planning the reform of nurse education. She explains how, as the NHS reforms proceeded, it became impossible not to conclude that nursing was considered insignificant by policy makers, medics and managers alike; it adapts to whatever circumstances are determined by others (Davies 1995: 46). Medicine relies upon the gendered nature of the lower status work done by para-medical groups, nurses, clerical and ancillary staffs, to maintain its position of professional privilege. Because nursing is seen in planning terms as subsidiary to the 'real' business of providing medical care, this has a knock-on effect in terms of the organisation of work on the hospital ward. Nurses are ancillary pairs of hands who deliver support and 'cover' the gaps in services: for the profession, 'the real and painful irony in this context is that there is no clear professional role at all' (Davies 1995: 151).

In 1986, the UKCC published its proposals for a new system of nurse training: *Project 2000: A New Preparation for Practice*. Training was to be dissociated from service delivery and take place in educational institutions rather than hospital schools of nursing; students were to receive funding through bursaries rather than wages and become independent of the employing authorities. This can be seen as a triumph for the professionalisers, and some analysts see the change in this way;[6] others view it as a renewal of the professionalising project.[7] Salvage claims that education and research play a key role in the professionalising project: research is developing a stronger philosophical and scientific base for nursing knowledge, substantiating the claim that nursing is a therapeutic practice, that care involves a holistic approach to the whole person and that the nurse/patient relationship helps the sick individual to mobilise their own resources to aid the healing process. She is, however, cautious in her assessment of these changes: 'Although New Nurses claim to be acting in patients' interests, they are also challenging medical domination and seeking higher status for themselves' (Salvage 1992: 14). Those in favour of Project 2000 envisage that it will enhance the development of professional practice, at the same time creating a fluid system of training that allows progression to different levels of expertise within the career structure. Others argue that nursing has chosen an educational model of professionalism that moves away from practical or vocational preparation. Sam Porter argues that Project 2000 has set the pattern for a small elite in nursing to gain status at the expense of the bulk of nurses who do the work and who will remain in a subservient position (Porter 1992: 724).

The problem of differentiating nursing from other groups with an interest in providing caring services is highlighted by the development of National Vocational Qualifications (NVQ) in Care, a development approved by the nursing profession in its negotiation of student status for Project 2000 trainees (Dalley 1993). Care services always utilise 'aids' but with exception of the Enrolled Nurse, until recently the formal preparation and assessment of health care assistants was not recognised. Warr (1996) argues that nursing is not a homogeneous profession – it is hard to propose a core set of key skills other than under a general heading of 'caring'; core units of the NVQ in Care testify to nursing's inability to monopolise on these. NVQs are a response to the demands of a market-led care industry that is re-evaluating the contribution of nurses who are no longer under the control of employing authorities while in training. General managers, not nurses, control the employment of health care assistants; nurses no longer have a strong role in planning and managing the service. Vocationally prepared staff, trained and assessed in many cases by managers, will not be 'nurses' but will share many facets of the caring role with nurses. Jeremy Warr points out that the vocational preparation of NVQ candidates is similar to the system of nurse training prior to the introduction of Project 2000; in an analysis of the effectiveness of level 3 NVQ support staff, it was found that the quality of care they provided was equal to and sometimes superior to that provided by junior grades of qualified nurses (Warr 1998). He argues that as NVQs develop levels 4 and 5 in Care, nursing needs to be sure of its quality contribution and cost-efficiency in the 'industry' of health care (Warr 1996).

Changes in the education and training of nurses and health care assistants have taken place against a background of crisis in recruitment; from the mid-1980s recruitment and retention of nursing staff again became a national issue. Between 1981–2 and 1986–7, the numbers entering basic nursing training fell by 29 per cent; of those accepted for training, 21 per cent failed to qualify or register or work in the NHS (Price Waterhouse 1988 in Walby et al. 1994: 22). A demographic time bomb had exploded; there was a sharp decrease in the size of the cohort available for recruitment at the very time that increasing numbers of elderly people stimulated the demand for nursing services. Pay was also a factor; staff nurses' salaries continued to lag behind those of other male-dominated public service professions such as the police and fire service.[8] By 1988, 40 per cent of nurses were earning less than the Low Pay Unit's threshold (Delamothe

1988 in Walby *et al.*, *ibid.*). Changing social expectations, political values and financial constraints put strains on a large, youthful workforce at a time when other, better-paid job opportunities were developing fast in other areas of the economy (Nicholson Lord 1988 in Owens and Glennerster 1990: 29). Although nursing was still a popular option for young women, it was at a disadvantage in competing for the declining numbers of young people in the age group that usually entered training.

By the early 1980s, the DHSS had delegated the task of organising nursing recruitment to an advertising agency, TBWA. The campaign launched in 1982 was markedly different from its predecessors; instead of emphasising caring, it stressed the intelligence required to become a qualified practitioner, using anatomical images of a heart and a brain and the tag line: 'What part of your anatomy makes you want to be a nurse? Your heart? Your head?'[9] The campaign won four major awards from the advertising industry, yet between 1982 and 1985 there was a marked decline in nursing's popularity as a career choice among young women and men and school leavers. An internal report on the campaign prepared by the Central Office of Information noted that although the campaign was, in its own terms, highly successful and acclaimed, the media's preoccupation with the decline of the NHS had produced a spate of negative imagery, fuelling fears of deteriorating conditions and low wages among potential recruits (Dickson 1987).

Some enterprising district health authorities responded to the challenge to improve recruitment by running their own campaigns at local level. Helen Richardson describes the initiatives undertaken by Northamptonshire which included commissioning an updated folder of fact sheets, a series of posters and a video that follows a group of students through their training. The initiative was launched with a cheese and wine evening for careers teachers and job centre staff, providing an informal occasion to discuss opportunities in nursing and counter negative perceptions. Part of the campaign aimed to attract older trainees: posters were placed in libraries and citizens advice bureaux; press releases were issued to local newspapers, radio and TV stations generating articles, radio interviews and local TV coverage of the campaign launch. The results were highly successful; the school of nursing filled its places for the year. Summing up the campaign, Richardson comments: 'By using marketing techniques employed by local competitors, we have ensured that we can hold our ground in the increasingly competitive workplace market' (Richardson 1988: 47).

Marketing nursing as a career choice in the late 1980s took place against a background of falling wages in real terms and a barrage of media criticism of worsening conditions within NHS hospitals. The government stepped up its funding for recruitment to four million pounds and commissioned a series of advertisements in national newspapers and magazines, followed by commercials on television that used real nurses rather than models. The advertisements contained the rather ambiguous wording 'What did you do at work today?' figured against typical office imagery such as the tabs of a filing cabinet, a piece of paper in a typewriter and a crossword puzzle. For the first time a recruitment campaign sought specifically to address those who had formed the staple supply of nursing labour since the beginning of the century – office workers and low-grade clerks. The nursing officer responsible for publicity strategies at the Department of Health, Patricia Collinson, claimed that it was the first attempt for several years to recruit actively rather than present a particular image of nursing (Vousden 1989a: 29). Staggered to run over several years, the campaign was criticised by some for 'presenting stereotypically dull and boring images' that did nothing to highlight the diversity of nursing and its rewards, or change people's perceptions of the profession (Tattam 1989: 22).

The strategy had some success in reaching its target group in an environment where equal opportunities policies presented obstacles to depicting nursing as a gendered profession.[10] For the first time a major recruitment campaign monitored and analysed how many of those who responded to the advertisements actually took up places in training, providing useful information about the sort of people choosing to become nurses. Some 30 per cent of enquiries were from respondents aged 17 or under, indicating a healthy response from the 'endangered species' of school leavers (Vousden 1989b); 86 per cent of all respondents were female; and the highest response came from the key target groups – women aged 16–24, men and women in this age group with five or more 'O' levels (GCSEs), and those likely to change jobs. It is difficult to quantify the effects of an advertising campaign with any degree of accuracy but it was estimated that at least a third of people who applied for a nursing course after receiving the information pack were influenced by the campaign and that there was a small improvement in the image of nursing amongst 16- to 24-year-olds (Vousden 1989b).

In contrast to the recruitment materials produced by the government, private health care companies such as BUPA consistently use images of female nurses on the front of their advertising leaflets and in their television adverts. The images are invariably of a white nurse in a traditional Sister's uniform often sitting at a desk, an image virtually identical to that used by the Nursing Recruitment Service in the 1960s. An image of feminine respectability is used to advertise private medical services arguably because it reassures purchasers of private health care that old-fashioned standards of excellence – embodied in the Nightingale image – are maintained in the private sector.

Amidst the general climate of crisis that has surrounded debates on the NHS, the crisis in nursing labour power has been an on-going focus of public concern with shortages in newly qualified nurses reported in the press in 1998 as approximating 8,000 per year.[11] Young people – and young women in particular – seem to be less interested in becoming nurses than in the past. A study of young people's perceptions of nursing as a career indicates that although nurses are admired for the work that they do, nursing is seen as physically demanding, low skilled 'dirty' work. Young people consider a career to be desirable if they admire what people do and seek to emulate those who do it; nurses are not envied and there is little about the nursing role that they aspire to or wish to emulate. Shift work and low pay are additional disincentives, fuelling perceptions of nursing as a low status occupation. Jane Hemsley-Brown and Nicholas Foskett describe these perceptions as a kind of snobbery; irrespective of the age, gender or social class of the research participants, nursing is perceived as a gender specific, low status service occupation that involves physical labour and a limited level of intellectual skill. These views are notably similar to middle-class views about the lower intelligence of nurses, doing chores, the discipline and poor pay in the post-war period. Of their total sample of more than four hundred young people in a range of educational settings,[12] only 6.6 per cent expressed an interest in nursing on the basis of doing a job that would 'help people'; young people of all ages, including a high percentage of 17-year-old girls, questioned why anyone would want to go to university to become a nurse. If they were going to go to university, they might as well attempt to become a doctor. Their knowledge about nursing was largely gleaned from parental attitudes and the influence of family, friends and the media, particularly television (Hemsley-Brown and Foskett 1999).

Romance in crisis

Television has become the principal mediator of knowledge and information to young people as well as providing a staple diet of entertainment. Television dramas, in particular, play an important role in representing gender relations and in showing how more egalitarian relations between different groups might be established and maintained.[13] Children's literature has entered a dialogue with a young readership familiar with television and, increasingly, computer games; fantasy, horror and science fiction are the preferred genres of choice, with occasional adventure series that feature 'emergency' scenarios. A survey of over 4,000 children found that for girls aged 11–16, the most frequently chosen genre is horror.[14]

Nurses rarely feature in books or magazines aimed at young people and the presence of nurses as central characters in films and romantic fiction has declined. A few career novels do still focus on nurses, such as the 'Point Nurse' series written by Bette Paul (1995, 1996),[15] and there are texts designed to inform readers about nursing as a career such as *Becoming a Nurse* by Angela Waring (1996)[16] and *A Day in the Life of a Nurse* by Carol Watson (1996).[17] Other books are published as tie-ins to popular

TV series such as *Children's Ward* (Granada 1995) and *Staying Alive* (LWT 1996) or pick up on popular TV themes, such as the 'Emergency' series by Lisa Rojany (1996) and the 'City Hospital' series by Keith Miles (1995): all of these texts foreground general nursing and/or hospital nursing.

Children's Ward: The Crash, written by Helen White and published by Puffin Books, is an issue-led text written to accompany the popular TV drama. The story focuses on a group of 'joyriders' whose theft of a car kills one of their gang and leaves another with serious mental impairment. Given the book's attention to young people's problems and its treatment of contemporary issues, the depiction of nurses and nursing has a decidedly old-fashioned ring – a *Sue Barton* book for our times. A young but fatherly doctor manages the medical care; his wife, formerly the ward Sister, works as a staff nurse and manages the care of their young son. Amongst the five nurses depicted in the text the auxiliary is an archetypal 'mother', and the Sister in charge, from the children's point of view, is something of a prim and starchy old maid until she becomes responsible for the care of a motherless teenager and romantically involved with his father. Two students, one male and one female, complete the nursing team. Nursing is depicted as a difficult, demanding job that requires constant tact and diplomacy, patience and a belief in the essential 'goodness' of those that are cared for. The differences foregrounded between the staff and children are those of class and age. The bourgeois values of the staff are a source of amusement and irritation to their young charges – they're just like teachers! Gender relationships are naturalised within the structure of care and race is not an issue, although the cover image depicts an ethnically diverse group of teenagers, effectively collapsing racial and class difference at the level of the plot.

In contrast, the 'Point Nurse' series presents nursing through a range of individuals undertaking their first year of training at a busy northern teaching hospital. Each book focuses on different aspects of nursing work through their psychological effects on six students, who have to come to terms with their own lives through the scenarios they encounter. Nick, a mature working-class student who spent much of his childhood in care, has to confront his own childhood neglect while working on the children's wards, and Barbara, a British-born Afro-Caribbean woman, faces her own grandmother's sudden death while on her geriatric placement. For Barbara, who has given up a career in accountancy with a prestigious City firm after realising she was their token black woman, nursing offers a future in managing a health service that she sees as in need of improvement. She aims to supplement her nursing degree with a further degree in business management in order to achieve her ambitions. Each of the six students is shown to have an aptitude for the different branches of nursing work, whether in the community or on the hospital wards, in mental health or paediatrics. The books challenge stereotypes of nurses and nursing; all the students have talents that could blossom in other fields of work but choose to be nurses because it offers the opportunity to use their other skills – as business managers, performers, producers and artists – within a therapeutic context. These trainees demonstrate care for the self and care for each other through friendship and emotional support, the sharing of food demonstrating and negotiating their cultural differences. In these books, nursing is shown to demand the whole self in willing service to an ethics of care and an ethics of responsibility, a positive image of equal opportunities in action.

Flames (1995), one of the books in the 'City Hospital' series by Keith Miles, features a team of five students who share a flat together: Mark and Bella are trainee nurses, Suzie is a student radiographer, Karlene a trainee physiotherapist and Gordy a medical student. Traditional hierarchies are very much in evidence in this book: senior nurses and tutors continue to be dragons, and when he meets the consultant 'Mark felt he was looking at a minor God' (1995: 103). The same doctor claims that Bella's pretty face is 'the best tonic for any young man' (1995: 106); the two students are treated as pairs of hands, moved around the hospital to wards where staff are short and expected to do menial tasks such as bed making. If the hierarchical, gendered relationships remain intact at the hospital, at home Bella is more than a match for Gordy and taunts him mercilessly. These books focus on the problems of young people's lives within a hospital context, rather than nursing lives *per se*, following the general drift of television fictions towards depicting hospital work as team work. Romance is an entertaining ingredient in all of these texts, but not a resolution to narrative problems.

Staying Alive (LWT 1996) was the only TV drama series in the 1990s to focus on the experiences of student nurses in training; a book written to tie in to the series closely follows the narrative of the TV text. Similarly to their counterparts in the 1950s and 1970s, the five nurses at the centre of the action are a representative selection of recruits but, following the more general currents of equal opportunities discourse, class difference is no longer an issue. Alice (Jessica Stevenson) is a weight-conscious 20-year-old in her third year; Mick (Susannah Wise) is an emotionally disturbed young woman of similar age; Cassie (Jenny Bolt), a mature female student, has taken up nursing to escape a violent marriage; Alan (Paul Higgins) is in his late twenties and married but cannot face up to the death of his young son. Kelly (Sophie Okonedo), the only black British student, is a good nurse but a stereotypically 'bad girl' who likes to party and have a good time. The 'naughty nurse' stereotype, formerly embodied in images of white working-class women, is displaced here on to the black female nurse. Lola Young argues that in films 'dirty' or transgressive sexuality 'is often displaced onto the racial Other ... in racist societies, no image is neutral or innocent of the past whether or not that past is acknowledged'

(Young 1996). In *Staying Alive* difference from nursing's feminine ideal is articulated as racial 'otherness' rather than class difference. Positioned as sexualised, Kelly bears the burden of representation of colonial history and its associative connotations, an interpretation reinforced by the irresponsible behaviour of her brother and his friends which places Kelly in conflict with an all-white nursing management who view her as a good nurse but a troublemaker. The double-faced nature of equal opportunities rhetoric is revealed in this imaginary encounter; on the one hand, there is a commitment to recruiting those ethnicised by the dominant culture, but on the other hand personality traits and behaviour are still depicted as a measure of 'difference' from middle-class white norms, as they were in the 1960s.

The male nurse Alan who becomes Kelly's lover is also a stereotype: a caring 'new man' who has difficulty coming to terms with his emotions, he is overtly and demonstrably heterosexual, perhaps to counteract stereotypical images of male nurses as gay. The interwoven plot lines revolve around the sexual and emotional lives of the students, their affairs with each other and the doctors and their relations with senior nursing staff. *Staying Alive* follows a general trend in TV drama of the 1990s in which the spectacle of sex is used to increase viewing ratings. Arguably, nurses fare no worse than other groups in this respect; doctors, male and female, in series such as *Cardiac Arrest* and the young lawyers in *This Life* receive similar treatment, but for images of nurses the connotative associations are significantly different. The focus on sexuality and depiction of sex acts fuels stereotypes of nurses, both male and female, as sexually promiscuous. Unlike medicine and law, where sexual behaviour between its practitioners is perceived as 'normal' amongst young people, revealing the sex lives of nurses tends to confirm deep-rooted anxieties about the 'natures' of those who nurse, serving only to confirm nursing's lower social status.

By the late 1970s, the popularity of Mills & Boon doctor/nurse romances was beginning to decline. Various attempts to re-invigorate readers' interest were attempted throughout the 1980s and early 1990s but the market did not recover, and they are now considered the least profitable of romantic sub-genres (Williamson 1998). In an attempt to revive falling interest from readers, in 1993 Mills & Boon re-titled their doctor/nurse romance series 'Love on Call'. Doctors were still considered an essential part of the formula, but there was greater flexibility in the female role; she could be a nurse, but other para-medical roles, such as occupational therapists, physiotherapists and radiographers were equally possible, with female doctors becoming more prevalent (Williamson 1998). In 1996, a further change re-titled the sub-genre 'Medical Romance'; the vast majority of these books focus on relationships between male and female doctors – nurses are no longer part of the romantic novel's medical formula.

The growth of the market for science fiction has provided potential opportunities for re-visioning the relationship between medicine and nursing, but analysts of science fiction find little that is optimistic here.[18] Future visions often re-negotiate the boundaries between gender, work and space, but the work of caring for the body remains invariably within a bio-medical paradigm of doctor-centred care; in the popular US TV series *Star Trek*, for example, the physical tasks of caring are managed technologically and a hologram of a male doctor provides reassurance and emotional support (Moody 1998).

Changes in the career opportunities available to young women have altered their aspirations; nursing no longer captivates contemporary readers as it once did. The fascination with medical science and the aspiration to become middle-class that sustained the doctor/nurse romance has also diminished; Williamson (1998) argues that in contemporary medical romances the frisson of desire demands a strong and independent female who can oppose the hero on the grounds of professional ethics. In the public imagination, nursing seems to be losing out to other groups in providing an image of ethical care: in the TV drama *Life Support* (BBC 1 1999), patient advocacy is in the hands of a professional medical ethicist and nursing relegated to a task-based activity.

Equal opportunities in crisis: medical drama[19]

In 1996, viewing figures for medical drama reached an all-time high in Britain, with some fifteen million viewers watching *Casualty* and thirteen million watching *Peak Practice*. In the US, *ER* topped the charts as the most popular drama in any category, while in Britain it became cult viewing on Channel 4, achieving viewing ratings in excess of four and a half million (Lawson 1996). The prevalence and popularity of emergency medical dramas suggestively indicates a continuing need for reassurance in our medical services. In the emergency scenario, at worst, doctors are seen to 'first do no harm' through any ill intent, and more importantly, they are shown to save lives successfully. Modernisation of the generic repertoire of the medical melodrama during the 1980s consisted of, on the one hand, extending the range of contemporary health issues to include Aids, rape, homelessness and drug-related incidents, and on the other a more spec-tacular iconography that graphically depicts the gore of accidents, injury and resuscitation. These changes were accompanied by a shift in focus away from the single figure of the doctor – from *Dr Kildare*, *Marcus Welby* and *Ben Casey* in the 1960s and 1970s – to the concept of the medical team in *Casualty*, *ER*, *Cardiac Arrest* and *Chicago Hope*. Within the medical team, women play doctor and men play nurse: the gendered division of labour in health care is shown to be shifting in line with sexual discrimina-tion policies that enable women to occupy professional roles traditionally monopolised by men, and men to engage in servicing roles traditionally occupied by women. This discourse is operative at two levels: in the institutional context of broadcast television, and within the formal dynamics of the melodrama as a realist text engaged with contemporary issues and debates. In institutional terms, the enactment of equal opportunities policies is visibly evident on the screen at the level of casting. 'Equal opportunity' is a central dynamic across a range of contemporary medical dramas, but, as I discuss in more detail below, the masculine vision of the professional ideal, apparently challenged by these shifts in representation, is invariably sustained.

On television, an on-going concern with and interest in the state of the nation's health was demonstrated in the early 1990s by the number of programmes that regularly depicted how the NHS was coping (or not) with changes in the organisation of health care delivery. Numerous documentaries charted 'a day in the life of' a hospital (*Jimmys, Children's Hospital, Great Ormond Street*), while other series, such as *Hospital Watch* and *The Pulse*, attempted to gauge the state of the nation's health care provision. Light relief from the climate of crisis was provided by situation comedies such as *Health and Efficiency* that lampooned the managers' attempts to rationalise service delivery as well as the doctors for their bumbling paternalism and gross inefficiency. Dramas of reassurance, both factual and fictional, became increasingly popular in the 1990s: from the reconstruction of sensational rescue scenarios in series such as *999*, verité documentary productions of the emergency services in action such as *Blues and Twos, Call Red* and US variants such as *Trauma* and *The Real ER*, to the fictional *Casualty, Cardiac Arrest, ER* and *Chicago Hope*, medical dramas spectacularise the doctor–nurse–patient relationship. These emergency encounters repeatedly assuage the crisis of confidence in medical care that numerous commentators claim is due to a breakdown in trust brought about by the health reforms.[20] Emergency dramas offer reassurance that, at the very least, doctors will 'first do no harm' and that, more often than not, they 'save' us through their repetitive re-staging of life-saving scenarios of resuscitation.

During the 1980s, British terrestrial television had to respond to demands for equality of opportunity by providing programmes of interest to marginalised viewing constituencies.[21] As a public service funded by the licence fee, the BBC has a responsibility to enact equal opportunities policies but, as in other areas of public life, institutional response has been uneven. The BBC responded to government demands opening up the broadcasting market by playing the equal opportunities card in support of public service broadcasting and enacting policy at the level of programme production.[22] Constraints were also placed on casting; it was no longer possible to discriminate openly on the basis of ethnicity. One result of these changes is that the image of nursing on television depicts a far more diverse range of characters that can be nurses than at any other time in the profession's history. No longer is nursing depicted as a white, middle-class, female-dominated profession; black and white, female and male, heterosexual and homosexual people from a variety of social class backgrounds and geographical localities occupy nursing roles. In other ways there is still plenty of ammunition to fuel arguments that, as a profession, nursing continues to be misrepresented. The most popular image of nursing and nurses is found in *Casualty* (BBC 1 1986 to date), a prime-time medical drama set in the accident and emergency unit of a large city hospital. General nursing continues to be the focus of media attention; specific programmes over the years have featured psychiatric care and children's nursing (*Children's Ward*, *Children's Hospital*), but within the context of programmes that are primarily focused on medicine and medical care. Few programmes feature nurses as central characters, although *Casualty*, foregrounds nurses and para-medics and their skills rather than the doctors, who are invariably shown as part of the medical team. *Staying Alive*, the only series in the 1990s to focus entirely on nursing students, adopted a similar approach to *Angels*, depicting the experiences of five student nurses as they progress through their training. Other medical dramas focused on the careers of young doctors, such as *Cardiac Arrest*, but this drama failed to attract a sufficiently large audience to warrant further series. Could this be, perhaps, because the leading medical character was female, acerbic and aggressive? This was not an image of a doctor that comfortably reassured viewers. Drama continued to be cheaper to import than to make at home; the usual diet of American medicals (in the 1990s *ER* and *Chicago Hope*) has accompanied broadcasting of the home product but significant differences between the two products continue, analysed in more detail below.

Casualty, began in 1986 with a bitter attack on government policy manifested in dramatic terms through an acute shortage of beds for critically ill patients. Was the timing co-incidental? Or was the health service perceived to have declined so rapidly that the BBC decided to risk producing a decidedly partisan drama in the interests of supporting one of Britain's best loved institutions? The writers claim that they wanted to make a campaigning programme; the outline for the initial proposal claimed: 'In 1945 a dream was born in the National Health Service. In 1985 that dream is in tatters' (Kingsley 1993). The programme initially blended several successful TV formats: three fictional streams, the medical drama, the soap opera and action adventure series, and two factual strands, the scientific demonstration programme and the campaigning political report. After a slow start and a storm of complaints, the formula proved highly successful at a time when BBC television was facing intense competition from its commercial rivals and the possible loss of funding from the licence fee.[23]

Medical melodrama traditionally stages the individual's sense of their own mortality and vulnerability when faced by the unpredictable onslaught of ill health and disease. This notion of helplessness, of feeling out of control of one's own body and its functions and needing to feel able to entrust that care and control to another, seems to lie at the heart of the genre's continuing popularity and fascination. In the 1950s, public faith in bio-medicine found its apotheosis and embodiment in the saintly demeanour, high moral character and good looks of the archetypal television doctor. This image added weight to analogies in popular fiction of doctors as god-like, larger than life characters with magical powers to create health and well-being. In the 1990s, hospital dramas re-worked this generic trope to embrace changes in the gendered identities of doctors and nurses. The shift was accompanied by a change in location from the domestic environ-ment of the hospital ward to the public spaces of the casualty department and the emergency room. Contact between doctor and patient/client, formerly envisioned as a process of consultation and confession, is minimised in favour of rapid action and visual spectacle; dramatic dramas of resusci-tation now constitute the focal point of the medical encounter on both sides of the Atlantic.

The 1980s saw major changes in the genre as it broadened its coverage of contemporary subject matter. In the USA, *St Elsewhere* grappled with the ethical issues presented by contemporary dilemmas such as euthanasia, Aids and rape. In Britain, *Casualty* opened on BBC 1 packed with topical issues and a bitingly critical attack on cuts in National Health Service funding that led to questions of 'bias' being raised in Parliament.[24] These new programmes, based on the dilemmas faced by over-worked and over-stretched hospital staff, seemed refreshingly topical, injecting a renewed sense of realism into the tired medical format. Women arrived on the scene as medics, men as nurses; issues of sexuality and ethnicity are acknowl-edged amongst the staff team, which replaces the single figure of the doctor at the centre of the action. Writers spent more time researching their stories; drawing on actual incidents and events, more simultaneous plot lines are woven into the narrative structure. Directors placed a renewed emphasis on visual realism that privileged authentic depictions of physical injury and a sense of immediacy conveyed by smaller, more mobile cameras and faster editing techniques. Karpf claims that the major change in 1980s dramas was to introduce the doctor as a human being, replacing the iconic waxworks of the Kildare mould with doctors who experience emotional and physical problems (1988a: 193). Re-situated as 'more like us', doctors came down from their pedestals to reveal their mortal feet of clay, shifting the focus of the narrative from professional conflicts to personal relationships and family crises. This trend continued into the 1990s in American melodramas such as *ER* and *Chicago Hope*, as well as in British variants such as *Casualty*, *Medics* and *Cardiac Arrest*. Within this framework of common shifts marked differences remain between British and American dramas, in part a result of their institutional production contexts and differing aesthetic traditions, in part due to the very different medical establishments they depict. A comparison of British and American programmes, focused on *Casualty* and *ER*, identifies how the genre has maintained key aspects of its traditional format in an attempt to retain the utopian sensibility of medical drama, whilst responding to an appetite for realism through their use of contemporary issues and visual strategies. At a glance, gender appears less of an issue in these dramas than formerly. Women are assimilated into the medical teams on an apparently equal footing with their male colleagues and the nursing and ancillary staff are as likely to be male as female.

Casualty began in 1986; since then it has seen many changes but the basic format remains the same, a blend of series drama and soap that concentrates on demonstrating complex medical procedures coupled with issue-based information. Every episode begins with an exposition, depicting the events that lead to a spectacularly realised accident and its immediate aftermath, demonstrating how the actions of irresponsible characters precipitate admission to the accident and emergency department. The educative impulse of earlier British dramas is retained through this format, but rather than informing the public about medical treatment, the series demonstrates how individuals are responsible for the misfortunes they bring upon themselves or cause others.[25] The on-going moral argument of *Casualty* is that injury and death are not just haphazard misfortunes but causally motivated by socially irresponsible individuals. The melodramatic trope, formerly personified in the patient as the unfortunate victim of disease or injury is displaced in *Casualty* on to frivolous citizens as villains, agents of death and disruption. A construction worker gambles away his family's house-keeping; hearing his horse lose on the radio, he loses his concentration, crushing his colleague with a chunk of concrete. The colleague dies. An alcoholic advertising man pours away his tipple when his girlfriend vomits blood after a drinking binge. A blind gypsy, suspicious of doctors and convinced her condition is hereditary, discovers after an accident that she only has cataracts. Moral messages of self-vindication validate bio-medicine's social mission; the effectiveness of a health service that constantly has to cope with civic irresponsibility is re-affirmed by spectacular demonstration while narrative resolution restores faith in the efficacy of bio-medical methods.

This moral element has often been counterbalanced by a preparedness to engage with issues of health service policy and funding, as well as professional antagonisms within the health care team. *Casualty* broke new ground in its representation of medical care, favouring a narrative structure where nurses and para-medical staff are given equal agency with doctors in the enactment of skills and expertise. Doctors in *Casualty* tend to be in the minority, with the focus of dramatic action centred on the para-medics and the nursing staff. Women inhabit the medical roles in (almost) equal numbers to men, but whereas the male doctors comfortably wear their professional personae irrespective of personal problems, females are shown experiencing a range of difficulties invariably associated with their gender and sexuality. Throughout its long history *Casualty* has shown an on-going preoccupation with the conflict between personal and working life. This is often played out through a traditional generic trope, the doctor/nurse romance, enacted with a contemporary twist. Charlie (Derek Thompson) is the nursing manager of the busy accident unit: *Casualty*'s longest serving cast member, he is known to regular viewers as a kindly and considerate man who nonetheless has problems coping with personal relationships. As nurse-in-charge he has to manage the day-to-day administration of nursing services, including recurrent problems of under-staffing created by cuts in the department's budget, and the emotional problems of staff, patients and relatives. Twelve years on since she first appeared as a senior house officer, Baz (Julia Watson) returned as the consultant in charge of the medical team and rekindled her romantic association with Charlie. Depicted as a competent and assured woman on the work front, her personal and emotional life is shown fraught with difficulties. Communication with Charlie suffers from a collapse of their inter-personal and professional worlds that he interprets as placing professional life before personal life at the expense of their relationship and the parenting of their young son. The issue of child care in an environment where both partners have to respond to emergency situations is graphically depicted in an episode in 1998 where Charlie, having failed to organise child care arrangements, is literally left holding the baby while his partner undertakes a heroic life-saving procedure. As a representation of a man in a traditionally female occupation, Charlie's position and status are revealed as subordinate to the dictates of professional hierarchy; situated as gendered female and inferiorly classed, he suggests the termination of a relationship which has tested his ability to cope with role reversal to the limits. Baz, faced with choosing between her career and her relationship, agrees to a separation, taking the child with her.

The problems of combining working life with single parenthood, explored in the early days of *Casualty* through the difficulties experienced by the female nurse manager Duffy, are foregrounded through another male nurse who has a child by a woman who is no longer his partner. In love with another man, she abandons the child to the care of Mark, who will now experience all the problems of single parenthood from a male nurse's perspective. But not only is Mark male, he is also black; *Casualty* has often focused on the long-term problems of incorporation faced by black male nurses in a traditionally white feminine role. Mark follows in the footsteps of other Afro-Caribbean nurses in *Casualty*, Clive King (George Harris) and Ash (Patrick Robinson), reflecting the programme's engagement with a broad spectrum of equal opportunities issues. Ash was depicted facing racism in his professional life through his fight for promotion to senior nurse and racism in his personal life created by parental opposition to his partnership with a white female student. During its long run *Casualty* has explored aspects of gendered identity and working relationships including the problems faced by gay male nurses, black male nurses and black female doctors. These shifts in representation, accompanied by an emphasis on the professional lives of nurses and para-medics, somewhat at the expense of doctors, would initially seem to enact a transforming vision of gender relations in health care. But apart from two notable exceptions (Duffy played by Catherine Shipton and Megan played by Brenda Fricker) male nurses have occupied much of the limelight in *Casualty*. Female nurses over the years have tended to conform to the more traditional stereotypes of young single students and older married women part-timers with children and domestic problems. In contrast, Charlie personifies many of the traits conventionally attached to male doctors: he too is a caring, compassionate man who privileges work rather than his personal life and reassures through his actions. By placing a male nurse at the centre of the action, the programme makers ensure continuity with medical melodrama's most familiar trope – the caring male medic – while meeting criteria for 'progressive' programming that demonstrates equal opportunities in action.

American series such as *Chicago Hope* and *ER* are known for their formal experimentation, yet both retain a strong melodramatic impetus that arises less from the moral imperatives of the storylines than from their continuing dependence on doctors as the personification of ethical and psychic motivations. The focus of discussion here is on *ER*, known for its hectic pace, the highly mobile use of the steadicam as it careers through the corridors, the unremitting use of high-tech equipment, its complex medical jargon and caustic humour. Less commented on, but equally important, are the use of muted colour tones that emphasise saturated colours, particularly red, low key lighting and hand-held camera work that creates a documentary look, and the melodramatic use of soft focus lenses accompanied by musical underscore at strategic points of emotional intensity. The combination of fast-paced, documentary technique with a romanticised aesthetic, a spectacular *mise-en-scène* of traumatic effect and strong character acting from the cast, provides a unique prescription for the ailing medical series, re-invigorating the form with a renewed sense of realist intensity yet leaving the traditional doctor-centred structure of medical melodrama intact.

Although the doctors in *ER* reveal their feet of clay, they are far from immobilised, their position at the apex of the health care hierarchy un-tarnished by the complexities of their private lives or the vicissitudes of an institutional structure where professional control is directly proportional to seniority. These doctors continue to be in charge, responsible for their actions and conscious of ethical dilemmas, presenting in a modern context all the attributes of their heroic forebears dispersed across a complex infrastructure of gendered and multi-racialised identities. Key to the recurring generic trope is the relationship between juniors and seniors, those who are responsible for passing on medical skills and expertise to younger, less experienced colleagues. Selection for positions of higher responsibility demands that skills are demonstrated to show that medical authority has its basis in the intellectual and physical skills of practice and experience, not in a spurious paternalistic authority. This gives the constant replay of life-saving procedures an added frisson, since each member of the medical team is present for the specific reason of career advancement. In this competitive environment, progress is constantly checked and monitored. Females jockey on equal terms with males for key positions in the surgical emergency teams, keen to notch up the requisite number of required procedures on their professional attainment records. The on-going conflict between the ambitious African-American Benton (Eriq La Salle), known for his rather surly nature, and Lizzie (Alex Kingston), a visiting female surgical lecturer from Britain, structures this dynamic around the gendered, racialised and national identities of the two protagonists. She plays on Benton's recent parenthood as an excuse to exclude him from an important surgical milestone, taking his place on the surgical team ostensibly on the grounds that he will want to spend time with his partner and their newborn child. Benton interprets this action as manipulation, leaving her to perform minor surgery alone and thereby breaking a professional code of practice in American hospitals which forbids any doctor to perform even minor surgery without the presence of a senior physician who is legally responsible. Coming from Britain, where independent action is given professional kudos, she is shocked to be severely reprimanded by a senior consultant and blames Benton for her *faux pas*.

Sponsorship is foregrounded as an on-going issue. Acting head of surgery Kerry Weaver (Laura Innes) is told by her boss to make further cuts in the departmental budget or lose his support on the hospital board. Her gender is a constant issue in her exchanges with male-dominated management; at a public meeting, her questions are dismissed through the use of a personal discourse of sexual attraction, diminishing her status far more effectively than her small physical size and damaged leg ever could. The masculine vision that underlies the concept of profession, as in earlier American medical dramas, is hidden and presented as gender-neutral. Nurses, physician's aids, social workers, secretaries and receptionists, mostly played by women, are busy background presences with single characters, such as nurse Carol Hathaway (Julianna Margulies) and physician's aid Jeanie Boulet (Gloria Reuben), singled out as token representatives of their respective trades. When the budget has to be cut, it is these 'non-essential' jobs that are the first to go, their workers seen as disposable commodities by a management keen to maintain the salary scale of the medical elite. This adjunct work, labour defined as 'feminine', is marginalised and rendered all but invisible, its value only accorded status by the acting female head of department who finds herself powerless to protect it. Kerry has to sack her friend and protégé, physician's aid Jeanie, and no amount of sympathy on her part can ameliorate the decision or save the friendship.

The masculine vision of profession is overwhelming in *ER* in comparison with its British counterpart. Professionalism itself is bureaucratised, the autonomy of individuals subject to constant monitoring and observation in a highly competitive, litigious environment. Public behaviour has to be guarded and monitored at all times. The strain of maintaining a professional veneer of objective compassion is revealed in the character of Dr Green (Anthony Eastwood) when sued by furious relatives for a violation of their civil rights: Green admits, in personal conversation, that his adrenaline caused him to behave inappropriately (emotionally) in a professional encounter. Loss of emotional control is equated with femininity and a lack of professionalism. Doctors in *ER* reveal their human flaws, but this humanisation is generally conducted through a focus on the ethics and responsibilities of maintaining the medical ideal. Personal life is inseparable from professional life, relationships with non-medical others destined to failure. The partnership between senior nurse Carol Hathaway and the philandering Dr Ross (George Clooney) is a cliché of the form.

ER is undoubtedly a richer world dramatically than *Casualty*, its ongoing series format creating the potential for both long-term problems and short-term conflicts. In a drama entirely centred on the medical staff, patients are little more than ciphers, nodal points for potential clashes of personal identity and professional ethics. Within this framework, *ER* engages issues of gender, 'race' and class as they pertain to or infringe on the professional ideal. In *ER*, there is no separate sphere of domesticity that offers relief from the constant pressure of professional demands, no 'feminine' vision that offers an alternative mode of thinking or being to the imperative of career success. The focus on the handsome, moody Dr Ross and his rather nerdish colleague Dr Green, the regular and most visible white male physicians, has made both men stars, a situation similar to that of Richard Chamberlain thirty years earlier who found international fame and stardom through his role as Dr Kildare. Both men are now playing kindly, compassionate men in Hollywood films, their star personas imbued with the ethos of their *ER* roles. Dr Ross and Dr Green may have come down from their pedestals and revealed their humanity, but in their enactment of American 'new man' sensibilities they perpetuate rather than dislocate the masculine vision of profession in US medical melodrama.

The personal is professional

Medical dramas on both sides of the Atlantic were privileged sites in the 1990s for re-staging the crisis of faith in health care as personal dramas of professional ethics. Within the public sphere, these dramas enact a masculine vision of medical care and ethical concern, combining concerns with fairness and social justice with responsibility for the care of others. The actual work of caring is still relegated to females, irrespective of their position as nurses or doctors: women rarely occupy senior positions of medical responsibility and when they do they are depicted as metaphorically and sometimes literally crippled (Kerry Weaver) by their femininity. Attempts to shift the gendered identity of medical protagonists in emergency dramas reveal the problems that lie at the heart of the sameness/difference disputes in the liberal feminist equal opportunities agenda. The melodramatic structures of popular series drama create heroes, villains and victims, whilst their content relies on contentious topical issues to fuel excitement, spectacle and moral dilemmas. Role reversal has to meet these conflicting dramatic demands, as well as broadcasters' needs for successful products. *Casualty* achieves these aims by altering the focus of the medical drama from doctors to nurses and para-medics, but by placing males at the centre of nursing action it retains an image of caring, sensitive masculinity. An episode of *Casualty* where Charlie saves Baz from the clutches of a kidnapper only serves to emphasise his heroic status while Baz, yet again, is shown to be weak and defenceless in spite of her high medical status. The doctor-focused *ER* also emphasises the vulnerability of its female medics with the result that it is those actors who play the most conventional roles in both *Casualty* and *ER* that have made their mark on popular consciousness.

Television is increasingly acknowledged as a mediator of public perceptions of professional identity. The on-going concern of the American Medical Association with their public image has kept questions of television influence on the research agenda, with the result that over the years a body of research has developed which attempts to analyse the effect of mediated images of medicine and medical practice on public perceptions of physicians.[26] Pfau, Mullen and Garrow (1995) argue that television is an important vehicle for secondary socialisation about professional roles irrespective of viewers' direct experiences. Leaving aside whether the cultivation theory that underlies their thesis is necessarily the most useful model of analysis in this context, there is a general belief amongst health professionals that these images influence at least some people's perceptions. In Britain, where questions of media influence are less of an issue on the research agenda, the Royal College of Nursing suspects that the portrayal of male nurses in *Casualty* has influenced an increase in male recruitment from under 10 per cent to more than 15 per cent of student applications in recent years. Pfau *et al.* propose that contemporary medical dramas illustrate a broader range of professional behaviours than individuals are likely to encounter through their direct experiences of medical consultation and treatment. Professionals manage their public performances, carefully controlling access to the non-public domain. Giddens sees this success in controlling the threshold between 'backstage' and 'frontstage' performance as 'the essence of professionalism', a precondition of maintaining trust as a form of faith (Giddens 1990: 86). The respect accorded to doctors is based on this trust, which derives from the control of specialised knowledge. Direct experience confines access to frontstage behaviours, but mediated experience potentially reveals backstage behaviour, with implications for trust (Pfau *et al.* 1995: 444). Contemporary medical melodramas take viewers behind the screens, revealing doctors' backstage behaviours, exposing the uncertainties of diagnosis, ethical dilemmas and the personal failings of those entrusted to heal. Pfau *et al.* conclude that there is an increased possibility of negative influence created by the revelation of 'backstage' behaviours that, in the longer term, may undermine trust in medical professionals. A gendered analysis of this research is highly suggestive, given that the revelation of 'backstage' behaviours corresponds with increased numbers of women depicted as medics and a heightened emphasis on the 'feminine' sphere of inter-personal working relationships and personal life. It is difficult not to conclude that the equal opportunities agenda is influencing public perceptions of medical power, a situation that American medical dramas in particular are re-negotiating through their use of traditional melodramatic textual structures.

The new fast-paced emergency dramas with their continuing emphasis on male actors at the centre of the action can be read as a re-assertion of medicine's professional ideal in the face of increasing social anxieties about the efficacy of bio-medicine and the ability of medical institutions to cope. In the face of such anxiety, demands for equality of representation are met by placing female actors in medical roles that undermine their professional status as autonomous 'frontstage' characters who manage their professional lives successfully. While the revelation of backstage behaviours can serve to humanise male professionals, females have yet to be given roles in medical melodrama where they embody the professional ideal. The irony for female doctors is that, in this the most caring of professions, they are placed in ambiguous relationship to their femininity. Depicting women as crippled, dependent and sexualised, contemporary medical melodramas serve only to confirm that for female health workers in nursing and medicine the road to equality in health care traverses a terrain somewhere between a rock and a hard place – a situation not too dissimilar to that faced in everyday life.

Carry on caring

Media formations of nursing identity in the 1980s and 1990s were subject to a discourse of equal opportunities that changed constructions of who can nurse but left the structural relationship between medicine and nursing intact. The climate of crisis that envelops public debate on the NHS is imagined as an emergency scenario in medical dramas, feeding a public appetite for spectacular images of the body in crisis that can only be saved by the medical team. Nurses, black and white, gay and straight, male and female, are depicted as skilled technicians and accomplished carers who work under conditions of unmitigated stress, a consequence of staffing and bed shortages created by budgetary constraints. Few other images of nurses are available. News and documentaries similarly focus on the hospital as the nexus of concern; financial constraints threaten medical excellence but nursing is left, amidst the chaos, to carry on caring. The climate of crisis within the NHS intensified after the introduction of the internal market; numerous documentary series in the early 1990s examined aspects of the effects of the changes on service delivery, such as *Operation Hospital* (C4 1992), *Cutting Edge* (C4 1992) and *The Pulse* (BBC 1 1994). Several series focused on the work of nurses, providing a platform for nurses to talk about their work: *Nurses* (C4 1992) examined a day in the life of a group of hospital nurses. Innovations in nursing practice and experimental projects focused on the autonomous delivery of care were presented on *The Pulse* (BBC 1 1994), and *Doctors and Nurses* (C4 1996) followed a night's work in a casualty department. The image of nursing depicted in these programmes was invariably that of the general nurse working in a hospital, reinforcing popular conceptions that this is what nursing is all about and where most nursing takes place. Within this context, the programmes emphasise a range of nursing skills from the everyday work of caring for large numbers of elderly, ill people and their relatives to the more technical aspects of managing sophisticated technological equipment. Nurses in these documentaries are frequently white and middle-class, with females outnumbering males; male nurses invariably address the problems of their image in a job where they are still seen as 'deviant' and often stereotyped as gay. Few programmes feature the experiences of black nurses although *Nurses* (BBC 2 1998), a documentary that followed the experiences of eight nurses undertaking the diploma at a Newcastle college, featured an Asian nurse, Martha Kumar, who acknowledged that she was a role model for other girls as Asian parents begin to accept women pursuing careers.[27]

How do nurses perceive their professional self-identity in this context? Research by Hoëpfl offers some indicative clues based on a small pilot study with six nurses. Hoëpfl used a repertory grid to provide a means of tapping social constructs which are not part of the stock of responses that can become the substance of interview data. The nurses were surprised by the discrepancy between their perception of the essential characteristics of their work and the extent to which other activities predominated in their day-to-day activities. This discrepancy was interpreted as indicative of the way the profession has changed and of increasing managerialism in the NHS. Their emotional attachment to their work appeared to be located in the tradition of 'service and dedication' to nursing as a vocation, their satisfaction gained from bedside nursing, but routine tasks were increasingly removing them from that ideal. It is not possible to generalise from such a small sample, but it indicates that studies of attitudes and values such as those by Ackroyd (1993) can contribute to an understanding of how organisational change is affecting the occupational perceptions of nurses.

In a follow-up study to the one above, Hoëpfl compared the professional attitudes and values of fifty nurses and fifty MBA students and clerical workers; for the female nurses the predominant career values were service, job security and lifestyle, for the men it was job security and service. For both genders, entrepreneurialism, competition, autonomy and independence and managerial concerns were low rated in comparison to the MBA students, who rated these values most highly. Female clerical workers had a similar profile to nurses, with an emphasis on service, job security and lifestyle. Perhaps this is unsurprising, given that female clerical and office workers often become nurses. Hoëpfl argues that the self-perception apparent in the production of the service identity appears to be devoid of competitive, entrepreneurial and control needs, a position that leaves nurses extremely vulnerable in a health service increasingly run by a competitive management ethos. These pilot studies indicate that however complex the issues which relate to the interpretation of the construction of professional identity by nurses, it is important to recognise the political implications of their core professional values and, within the current climate of health care, an increasing susceptibility to exploitation (Hoëpfl and Hallam 1995).

The correlation of self-perceptions of what constitutes a professional or 'proper' nurse with a personal conceptual framework founded on vocational values of service to the patient may change as the nursing profession attempts to re-mould itself to fit the market model in health care services.[28] In the past, differences between the competing power groups in the profession were somewhat tenuously held together by the professionalisers' control of a national training curriculum that included a heavy dose of moral education. In contrast, the modern nursing curriculum is shaped by the academic demands of the higher education system. These changes will have fundamental effects on nurses' self-perception as the current generation of educators and managers pursue a combined approach of academic study with a less rigorous practical training. Changes in discourse, away from notions of 'serving the patient' to providing 'care management facilities' for clients, are indicative of a less 'hands on' approach that will increasingly place the care of patients, particularly the elderly and incurable, in the hands of health care assistants and 'nurse's aids'.[29] These new discourses of nursing will percolate through the personal, professional and public imaginations during the next decade or so, as one generation of nursing leaders is replaced by another. It remains to be seen whether these emergent groups will succeed in re-shaping the rhetoric of 'tender loving care' that still cloaks much of nurses' work into a discourse that gives economic and intellectual value to the intimate work of caring intellectually, emotionally and physically for a sick person. Such a move will be necessary to ensure not only that high standards of nursing care are safeguarded for the patients/clients of the future, but that nursing skills and knowledge are recognised as essential and valuable assets in a society where cure is necessarily finite.

NOTES

INTRODUCTION

1 In her analysis of the social formations of class and gender, Skeggs (1997) emphasises how we are positioned differentially in terms of cultural capital. This is not just a question of being born with or without money, but of how our life chances, as members of social groups, are determined by how we construct our social identities in relation to 'normalising' discourses such as, in this case, the rewards to be gained by adopting (or not) the appearances and behavioural modes of femininity.

2 The peace camp was established in 1982 by women protesting at the housing of cruise missiles armed with nuclear war-heads at an American military base in Berkshire, England. The campaign and the encampment lasted until 1994 when the missiles were finally removed; the women at the camp survived police aggression, demonisation in the media and resistance from local landowners, the military and the police. For an account, see Young (1990) and for an analysis of the mediating role of television and the press see Couldry (1999).

3 Strategies are often conceptualised as the tools of official action and organised resistance; tactics are often seen as more anarchic, localised responses to unbearable circumstances. See Skeggs (1997) for a more detailed account.

4 See, for example, Stanley (1990a) for a sociological perspective, Skeggs (1995) for a cultural studies approach and Probyn (1993) for a theoretical account.

5 See, for example, Patton (1987), Burgess (1988), Strauss and Corbin (1990) and Bryman (1992). For a feminist ethnographic account of the relationship between self, work and knowledge see A. Williams (1990).

6 See, for example, Bell and Roberts (1984), Kreiger (1991), Stanley (1990a) and Shields and Dervin (1993).

7 For a more detailed discussion of gender and language and its relationship to structures of knowledge and power see, for example, Cameron (1985).

8 For accounts of Agnes Jones's work see F. B. Smith (1982), Baly (1986) and Dingwall, Rafferty and Webster (1988).

9 For an unusual attempt to situate psychoanalytic subject formation socially and historically using the methods of audience research, see Stacey (1994).

10 For a discussion of the debates on feminist uses of Foucault see, for example, Drummond and Quinby (1988) and McNay (1992).

11 Other examples of studies of female subject formation that take a generational approach are McRobbie and Nava (1984), Heron (1985), Steedman (1986), Jordan (1990), Press (1991), S. Douglas (1995).

202

12 Skeggs (1997) makes a similar point in her analysis of formations of class and gender.

13 See, for example, studies by Kalisch and Kalisch (1982a), (1982b), (1983) and (1987).

14 The only other interviews of this period in the National Sound Archive are the product of research sponsored by the Royal College of Nursing.

15 The principal acts are the Equal Pay Act (1970), the Sex Discrimination Act (1975) (amended), the Race Relations Act (1976), the Equal Pay amendment regulations (1983), the Sex Discrimination Act (1986), and the Disability Discrimination Act (1995).

1 IMAGES, IDENTITIES AND SELVES

1 Dingwall argues that Nightingale provided the evidence that her class really did care for ordinary soldiers, but the reality was that most of the caring work was done by those who had always done it – soldiers' wives and orderlies. 'What changed was the moral significance of the work; it became dominated by the values of the ladies and they took the credit for it' (Dingwall *et al.* 1988: 47). The promotion of Nightingale in her own time and subsequently has eclipsed the contribution of other women of different backgrounds and races to the care of the wounded in the Crimea. See, for example, Alexander and Dewjee (eds) (1984) *Wonderful Adventures of Mrs Seacole in Many Lands*, and J. Williams (ed.) (1987) *An Autobiography of Elizabeth Davis. Betsy Cadwaladyr: A Balaclava Nurse.*

2 Nursing historians such as Abel-Smith (1975), Baly (1980 and 1986), Davies (1980), Dingwall, Rafferty and Webster (1988) and Maggs (1983) tend to underestimate the power value of whiteness in constituting the discursive formations of modern professional nursing perhaps because it is so obvious we tend not to think about it; but, as Vron Ware (1992) argues, the apparent neutrality of whiteness does the most violence to those who are excluded from the terms of its address.

3 Stephen Lawrence was a young black male who died as a result of a racial assault in London in 1992. His murderers were never brought to justice, in part because of racist attitudes within the Metropolitan police force who were accused of institutional racism by a committee of public inquiry that published its findings in 1999. In response to these accusations, the Labour government vowed to eliminate institutional racism in all public service institutions. Institutional racism is sustained because of a lack of commitment within organisations to tackle structures that perpetuate racist practices. On the question of racism in nursing in the NHS see, for example, Beishon, Virdee and Hagell (1995).

4 This incident at the Annual General Meeting of the RCN was reported in the *Nursing Times.*

5 Salvage makes a similar point in her analysis of nursing's public image (Salvage 1985). It is disheartening to find how slow the pace of change has been on this particular issue.

6 Discourse is used here to mean a system of representation that is socially constructed to circulate coherent meanings about a specific social practice. Discourses are ideological insofar as they serve the interests of the group in society that generates them, naturalising coherent meanings into 'common sense', but they are not conspiratorial or 'produced' by individual authors or

speakers. Discourses are socially produced and often institutionalised ways of making sense of a topic; they construct a collective sense of social identity as we speak and write them. In this sense, they often reveal the collectively unconscious structures of the social formation. (See, for example, Fiske 1987: 14–15.)

7 For a feminist approach see, for example, Monteith (1986) and Shields and Dervin (1993).

8 See, for example, Brown and Jordanova 1981: 389–99.

9 Most commentators and analysts have focused on the class relationships between the working-class women who performed the bulk of nursing duties and the 'ladies' who took managerial and organisational responsibilities for their work. See, for example, Gamarnikow (1978 and 1991), F.B. Smith (1982), Simnett (1986) and Dingwall et al. (1988).

10 McClintock (1995) argues that the self-definition of the middle classes and the cult of domesticity were central to maintaining the imperialist project: categorisations of race were interlocked with those of class through the generic definition of 'dangerous classes'. (See Skeggs 1997: 5–12.)

11 Wendy Webster (1998) makes a similar point using this quote from George Sims, *How the Poor Live:* 'In these pages I propose to record the result of a journey into a region which lies at our own doors – into a dark continent that is within easy walking distance of the General Post Office. This continent will, I hope, be found as interesting as any of those newly-explored lands which engage the attention of the Royal Geographic Society – the wild races who inhabit it will, I trust, gain public sympathy as easily as those savage tribes for whose benefit the Missionary Societies never cease to appeal for funds' (quoted in Keating 1976: 65–6). The social explorers journeyed to urban areas in Northern England and the East End of London – areas populated by poor whites, some of whom were immigrants. These were also the areas targeted by early health visitors; see Davies (1988).

12 This phrase continued to reverberate throughout the inter-war period; Lord Reith, head of the BBC, and John Grierson, founder of the British documentary film movement, saw their role as cultural missionaries seeking to install middle-class tastes in the 'jungles' of the north.

13 Dyer (1997) points out that associations between spirituality and cleanliness are prominent in the writings of Protestant reformer Martin Luther (1997: 75). Nightingale was a Unitarian with a strong sense of personal vocation that placed a Protestant emphasis on the importance of performing Christian deeds (Dingwall et al. 1988: 37).

14 In his renowned lecture of 1931, Freud uses the metaphor of the 'dark continent' to represent female sexuality. Sigmund Freud (1931), 'Female Sexuality'.

15 Nightingale, like many upper-class women of her day, wholeheartedly supported colonialism; in 1859, she contributed a report to the Royal Commission appointed to investigate sanitary conditions in the Indian army. See Poovey 1989: 194–6.

16 Nightingale's views on the working class were not dissimilar to those of Engels (1844/1958) who noted that they were a 'physically degenerate race, robbed of all humanity, degraded, reduced morally and intellectually to bestiality' (p. 33) and 'a race wholly apart' (p. 361). (Quoted in Skeggs 1997: 5.)

17 See, for example, critiques of the representation of women in films by Haskell (1974), Mulvey (1975) and de Lauretis (1987); in the media more generally see Davies, Dickey and Stratford (eds) (1987); in the fine arts see Betterton (1987).

18 Laura Mulvey (1975) argues that this imaginary figure of woman is always constructed with the pleasure of male viewers in mind. For a development of this view in relation to the narrative structure of fictions, see Theresa de Lauretis (1987).

19 See Melosh (1984), Banks (1988), Fiedler (1988) and Hunter (1988) for studies of nurses in American literature and popular fiction.

20 In 'The invisible woman', Ann Preston (1990) analyses the image of nursing in a selection of women's magazines aimed primarily at young North American readers between 1967 and 1987 in order to ascertain whether the images of nursing in publications such as *Seventeen*, *Ladies Home Journal* and *Working Woman* present nursing as an interesting and attractive career choice. She concludes that nursing is 'curiously absent from the list of professions featured by the magazines most likely to influence young women while they are making their career decisions'.

21 For an analysis of images in the popular press see Dunn (1985).

22 See the *Report of the Committee on the Training of Nurses for the Colonies* (1945) which states that training is for supervisory and administrative posts.

23 Class analysis in nursing history since the nineteenth century tends to focus on psychiatric nursing rather than general nursing. See, for example, Carpenter (1978 and 1980) and for an account of nursing and trade unionism Hart (1994). For an account of women in trade unions, see Drake (1983). For a more recent class critique of the professionalising project in nursing see Porter (1992). Interestingly, the critique of class tends to come from male nurses, perhaps because many male nurses entered the profession from the 'lower' status field of psychiatric nursing. See subsequent chapters for a more detailed discussion.

24 Unpublished report, Department of Health (1966).

25 Throughout this period men considered nursing a choice of career suitable only for their daughters, not for their sons.

26 For an account of working-class female aspirations in the post-war period see Steedman (1986).

27 Personal communication, Mr R (1992). See subsequent chapters for a more detailed analysis of these issues.

28 Marsh and Willcocks (1965) in MacGuire 1969: 145; National Opinion Polls Ltd (1966) in *ibid.*: 151.

29 Charlotte Brunsdon (1991 and 1993) has discussed the development of a division between 'feminists' and 'women' and the problems arising in research and teaching from the conflicting desires of women (for femininity) and feminists (to transform ordinary women into feminists). With the increasing intellectualisation of feminist politics, feminist academics, in defining the ordinary woman as 'not me', have come to define themselves not only as 'not feminine' but also as 'not ordinary women'. For a discussion, see Hallam and Marshment (1995a).

30 For a more detailed discussion of this point, see Lawler (1991).

31 See, for example, the RCN's (1992) collection of nurses' work experiences.

32 The decision to focus on women was a personal one, initially based on my desire to explore how the women who trained me perceived their nursing identities.

33 For early examples of this approach see L. Anderson (1980), Jelinek (1980) and Gardiner (1981).

34 For approaches to the use of case studies and life histories see Hankiss (1981), Thompson (1981), Geiger (1986), Platt (1988) and Kreiger (1991).

2 THE POPULAR IMAGINATION

1 In telephone interviews conducted with four retired senior nurses, all commented that positive images of nurses on the big screen had a marked effect on recruitment. There is no researched evidence of this relationship between feature films and recruitment, but for an account of the effects of using recruitment films in the school context see Jeffery (1950).

2 Cognitive theories of textual interpretation foreground engagement and alignment with characters as processes that encourage empathy and secure moral allegiance. For a more detailed discussion of alignment and moral allegiance in popular films, see 'Discerning viewers' in Hallam with Marshment (2000).

3 See, for instance, Murphy (1983 and 1989); MacNab (1993).

4 Janet Thumim's research reveals that Hollywood films were the most popular films at the box office throughout this period (1992).

5 For a detailed account of female scriptwriters in Hollywood, see Lizzie Francke (1994).

6 It was released soon after the report on nursing produced by the Athlone Committee (1939). The report was commissioned after sustained pressure from trade unions with nursing members forced the government to re-evaluate pay and working conditions; see Hart (1994).

7 A detailed account of the novel is provided in Chapter 4.

8 Athlone Committee (1939), Maggs (1983).

9 *Mise-en-scène* is a French term used to refer to the pictorial and staging aspects of cinema.

10 Marian McMahon (1991) deconstructs this imagery in her experimental film *Nursing History* (1989) which analyses home movie footage of family weddings and her nursing graduation.

11 Richard Dyer argues that photographic and filmic technology has developed around lighting for whiteness. Photography, as a medium, developed in response to demands from white bourgeois clients for portraits of themselves and their families. Both film stock and lighting technology have developed around lighting the white face, creating a culture of practice and assumptions about 'beauty', 'glamour' and 'truthfulness' that were adopted and adapted by the movie industry. See 'The light of the world' in Dyer 1997: 82–144.

12 The use of character-centred biography to depict historical events in popular cinema perpetuates common-sense ideologies that individuals are the motor force of history rather than underlying structural forces. See Roland Barthes (1973) for a detailed analysis of the 'naturalising' power of myths.

13 See, for example, *Saturday Night and Sunday Morning* (Reisz 1961) and *A Kind of Loving* (Schlesinger 1962). John Hill (1985) argues that these films perpetuate conventional representations of working-class life through a focus on sexuality defined by the male characters.

14 This is an estimate based on the reprint dates of popular series and the introduction of new series rather than on reading figures, which are impossible to estimate.

15 These include the *Bunty Brown* books written by Barbara Wilcox and published by Oxford University Press 1940s, this edition 1959; the *Nurse* series written by Paula Deal, published by Arthur Barker Ltd, London (dated edition 1963); the *Sue Barton* books written by Helen Dore Boylston, published in Britain by Bodley Head from 1939 to 1959, reprinted by Knight Books (1968, 1981); the *Jean* series written by Doreen Swinburne, published by Collins (dated editions 1957, 1958, 1960, 1970); the *Nurse* series written by Constance M. White, published by Collins late 1950s and in paperback by Dragon 1970 and

1988; the *Cherry Ames* series written by Helen Wells and Julie Tatham, first published in America in the early 1940s, published in Britain by World Distributors Ltd in the late 1950s, reprinted several times until 1963. Dates of publication are subject to variation in different editions of the same text; in some cases, no publication dates are specified. With thanks to Dr Alice Kiger for her help in compiling this information.

16 Estimate based on the numbers of reprints and publisher's estimate of world-wide availability.

17 *Sue Barton: Student Nurse* was reprinted in Britain for the twelfth time in 1960.

18 The last edition of the *Sue Barton* stories I have found was published by Knight Books in 1981.

19 This edition, 5th reprint, 1959.

20 The books were frequently presented as school or Sunday school prizes; many of them contained a presentation certificate glued to the flyleaf.

21 Tinkler argues that magazines and popular literature construct and manage adolescence as a period of transition between childhood and adulthood. Adolescence is the product of late nineteenth- and early twentieth-century initiatives which institutionalised a prolonged period of dependency of young people on the family, facilitated by the extension of compulsory schooling and restrictions on child labour. See Tinkler 1995: 2–8.

22 For a development of this point see Hallam (1996).

23 *Sue Barton: Visiting Nurse* is dedicated to an American foremother, Lavinia Duck, founder of the Henry Street Clinic and its team of visiting nurses. I am grateful to Deborah Philips for drawing this to my attention: see Philips (1998).

24 Reiteration refers to the reproduction of representations through self-reference; it reinforces ideas and concepts and 'naturalises' them as common sense. It is argued here that reiterations serve ideological agendas that are always culturally and historically specific. For a development of the argument on reiteration and ideology, see Butler (1992).

25 See, for example, the descriptions of Marianne, a 'waif' from the slums transformed by Sue into an amusing variation of nursing's feminine ideal in *Sue Barton: Visiting Nurse*.

26 The literature on nursing and the military is extensive: see, for example, Cynthia Enloe (1983), Anne Summers (1988).

27 R. Williams (1963, 1977) analyses patterns of change in mood and atmosphere that can be traced in popular literature.

28 The cinema audience declined in the 1950s as people moved out of the inner cities to the suburbs and television increased in popularity. Between the post-war period and 1961 audiences declined from around 900–1,000 million visits a year to 515 million. For a discussion of these changes see Docherty, Morrison and Tracey 1987: 16–29.

29 The new wave of interest in the *Carry On* films in the 1990s is reflected in their presence in video shops, the popularity of Barbara Windsor (heralded as a national institution) and the considerable attention they are given in a range of academic work.

30 On the 1950s, see Lewis (1992); on the New Look see Hopkins (1963). For a detailed account of the relationship between fashion, film and femininity in British cinema see Cook (1996).

31 Mulvey (1975) analyses the relationship between the spectacle of femininity (women's 'to-be-looked-atness') and the male voyeuristic gaze as an integral element of the interplay between narrative pleasure and desire, claiming that this relationship reveals the deep-rooted structures of the patriarchal imaginary.

32 Propp analysed over 100 Russian fairy stories and found a common narrative in which the hero is invariably on a quest which ultimately ends in winning the hand of the one he loves. See 'Morphology of the folk tale' in Ashley (1989).

33 For an account of these experiences see Beryl Gilroy's autobiography *Black Teacher* (1994).

34 *Till Death Us Do Part*, writer Johnny Speight, BBC 1 1966–8, 1972, 1974–5.

35 This is particularly true for romances situated in exotic locations, where descriptions of the landscape are often used as a metaphor for female sexual passion. See, for example, the cover blurb on *Doctor Divine* (Sheila Burns, Pan Books, 1966): 'When ambition beckoned James to Africa, sudden opportunity allowed Dolores to follow her heart to the wild veld ... Beneath sultry skies Dolores found a dark world of witchdoctors, spells, and violent storms that mirrored the emotions in her own heart.' For a detailed critique of the racialised implications of this metaphor see L. Young 1996: 38–55.

36 For an exploration of the social construction of the 'normal' healthy body as racially coded white see Gilman 1985 and Dyer 1997.

37 On the racialised discourse of 'miscegenation' see Young 1996: 84–114, Dyer 1997: 35–6 and Webster 1998: 47–52.

38 In the late 1980s, news stories of babies dying for the want of nurses trained in intensive care procedures created a similar furore.

39 Julia Smith was one of a minority of women of her generation to achieve a distinguished career as a television producer.

40 These changes are often referred to as 'the male nurses' charter' because they favoured a male career structure within the profession (Davies 1995).

41 One result of this consciousness was the formation of the Public Image of Nursing Campaign (PINC) which aimed to monitor the representation of nursing in the media. See Salvage (1983a).

3 THE PROFESSIONAL IMAGINATION

1 Despite the eventual passage of the Nurses Registration Act in 1919, a number of analysts conclude that it marks, paradoxically, the failure of nurses' professional project and a significant defeat for the registrationalists. The Act ensured that the central statutory body, the General Nursing Council, far from being an autonomous decision-making body, was subject to government approval and veto. See Dingwall *et al.* (1988), Witz (1992).

2 See, for example, the National Board for Prices and Incomes investigation (1968) in the Briggs Report (1972).

3 Pavey's history covers the development of nursing from an art, to a vocation and then a profession, and tends to concentrate on great people as the movers of history rather than on government policy or economic determinants (Pavey 1938). She is one of the historians that Abel-Smith is rather critical of in his treatment of nursing history.

4 For a more detailed discussion of gendered conventions in fine art see, for example, Betterton (1987).

5 Portrait photography at this time tended to be based on notions of classical composition found in fine art. For a more detailed discussion of the ideological implications of photographic portraiture see Jo Spence (1986).

6 The Athlone Committee 1939; its recommendations closely reflected those of the TUC charter. See Dingwall *et al.* 1988: 103.

7 Summarising the research into recruitment and attrition between 1940 and 1969, Jillian MacGuire concluded that highly qualified recruits were over-represented in intakes to schools of nursing attached to teaching hospitals; those with the lowest levels of academic attainment were found in disproportionate numbers in schools attached to non-teaching hospitals (MacGuire 1969: 56).

8 See, for example, Houlison (1946) in MacGuire 1969: 142–3; Lee (1959) in *ibid.*: 144–5; and Petrie and Powell (1951) in *ibid.*: 156–8.

9 See, for instance, Cross and Hall (1954) in MacGuire 1969: 168–9; Knight (1965) in *ibid.*: 177–8; and Liverpool Regional Hospital Board (1965) in *ibid.*: 178–9.

10 For a detailed discussion of the exclusion of particular groups of women health workers from female professionalising projects in nursing and midwifery see Ehrenreich and English (1973); on asylum workers see Carpenter (1980).

11 From its inception, the GNC was always a potential instrument of the state; according to Witz, 'nurses were tightly constrained within a state–profession relation within which they were the weaker partner, as well as within the employment relation between hospitals and nurses and the inter-professional relation between doctors and nurses' (1992: 165).

12 *Picture Post* pioneered the development of documentary photography in Britain in the 1930s through location-based action shooting. For an account of these developments see, for example, John Taylor (1982).

13 The King's Fund has always had a close association with these hospitals – St Thomas's (the original home of the first Nightingale School of Nursing), St Bartholomews (Barts), and Guys are perhaps the most famous – protecting and promoting their interests.

14 *Diana* was an updated version of the successful *Bunty* and *Judy* format; it included photographs of pop stars alongside more traditional stories of female heroism, some of which were produced as photo-narratives.

15 Government social survey (1968) 'Young School Leavers: An Enquiry for the Schools Council'.

16 Some commentators estimate a much lower figure; for example Morton-Williams and Berthoud (1971) suggest that overseas nurses formed 9 per cent of the hospital nursing population.

17 The Report of the Committee on the Training of Nurses for the Colonies recommended that 'Colonial Girls should be encouraged to take their general training in their own territories or groups of territories and should come to the United Kingdom or the Dominions mainly for post-registration courses. It is realised, however, that for some time a number of Colonial girls will wish to come to this country for their general training; such training should be the same as that given to nurses in this country who propose to go to the Colonies and should be followed by the special Colonial course mentioned above' (1945: 28).

4 THE PERSONAL IMAGINATION

1 Marsh and Willcocks (1965) in MacGuire 1969: 145; National Opinion Polls Ltd (1966) in *ibid.*: 151.

2 Reprinted in 1956 and 1957; this edition 1957 (Penguin).

3 Reprinted five times, 5th edition 1963; this edition 1957 (Pan Books).

4 Most of those interviewed wished to remain anonymous, some expressing concern that to reveal their identity may result in professional reprisals.

5 Irish nurses were subjected to racial stereotyping in the 1930s and 1940s; by the 1950s English attitudes were arguably slightly less bigoted but they were still refused training in many former voluntary and teaching hospitals; see, for example, Starkey 1994.

6 *Playboy*, for example, has regularly featured nude images of young women who claim to be nurses.

7 Richard Dyer points out that Joel Kovel identifies the importance of dirt in the writings of the Protestant Martin Luther in the late Middle Ages; what emerges is a disdain and disgust for the body: 'the body is dirty; what comes out of the body is especially dirty; the material world corresponds to what comes out of the body, and hence it is also especially dirty' (Kovel 1970: 132 quoted in Dyer 1997: 75).

8 It was, of course, the male body that was the ostensible cause of concern, but there was also a worry about the 'unnaturalness' of female body contact and possible connotations of lesbianism; see Lawler (1991).

9 On nurses and sexuality, see Salvage (1987a) and Lawler (1991).

10 For accounts of lesbian lives see, for example, the Lesbian History Group (1989) and Snape, Thompson and Chetwynd (1995).

11 For a 1970s account of 'good' and 'bad' behaviour amongst student nurses training in an American context see Kreuger (1978).

12 Helen Evers (1981) provides an important analysis of the differential treatment received by elderly male and female patients in long-stay geriatric wards that expands K. Williams' (1978) concept of custodial ideology.

13 Dickens' attitude to popular culture is typical of her class at this time; establishment values promoted realist aesthetics, typified in the first two films Dickens scripted. For a more detailed account of the relationship between realist aesthetics and liberal humanist politics see John Ellis (1996).

14 The same sentiment underlies many of the conclusions of the Briggs Report and is still echoed by those who maintain that nursing is misrepresented, conveying a 'false image' of nursing to a gullible public.

15 In her autobiography Andrews, now known as a best-selling author of doctor/nurse romances, describes how she was encouraged to write lighthearted, romantic fiction rather than serious novels.

16 See Stein (1967) on the doctor/nurse game and the updated discussion in Stein *et al.* (1990).

17 For a detailed account of training in these hospitals, see Pomeranz (1973).

18 In a report commissioned by the RCN in 1993 to examine the profile, attitudes, career expectations and employment opportunities of nursing students, gender, age, marital status, educational background and previous experience are significant variables but race and ethnicity are absent categories, perpetuating the invisibility of black and ethnic minority nursing students. See Seccombe, Jackson and Patch (1995).

19 In an analysis of the social construction of whiteness (Frankenberg 1993) white interviewees link the power of white culture with the privilege of not being named; whiteness is an unmarked or neutral category that names other people as 'others' and other cultures as 'cultural'. 'White culture had a great deal of power, difficult to dislodge from its place in white consciousness as a point of reference for the measuring of others. Whiteness served simultaneously to eclipse and marginalise others' (1993: 197).

20 For a more detailed discussion of the methodological and interpretative problems of this approach see Hallam (1999).

21 For a more detailed discussion of the power relations inscribed in the interview process see Edwards (1990). This work stands in stark contrast to earlier

feminist accounts of the interview process where gender is seen as a significant equaliser in same-sex female interview situations (for example, Oakley 1980).

22 The interviews pre-date the publication of the Department of Health's research into 'the experiences of nursing and midwifery staff belonging to ethnic minority groups in the NHS' conducted by the Policy Studies Institute (Beishon, Virdee and Hagell 1995).

23 A study by Iganski, Mason, Humphreys and Watkins (1998) questions this thesis; an analysis of recruitment data collated to evaluate implementation of equal opportunities by the English National Board for Nursing, Midwifery and Health Visiting indicates that black (African diasporic) applicants as a group are over-represented compared with the representation of groups in the population as a whole. What is revealed is that black (Asian diasporic) groups are significantly under-represented.

24 Black labour was used extensively to provide cleaning and domestic services in hospitals in London and the south. See Doyal *et al.* (1981) and Doyal (1985).

25 In my own set (early 1970s) a colleague became engaged to a doctor before completing her training. She was called to the Senior Nursing Officer's office and asked to discontinue her relationship.

26 In 1996 Nurse Nidir Firdous was awarded £50,000 compensation from her NHS trust for racial harassment after three years of unfair criticism, demotion and suspension by her employers. Five black nurses from Coventry were awarded £35,000 compensation from their trust after personality tests were used to justify downgrading (Mensah 1996).

27 Davies argues that this sense of commitment but frustration with the conditions under which nursing is done is due to a system that undermines the confidence of the nurse, restricts the contribution she can make, and creates a constant questioning about the quality of care that is being delivered (1995: 91–5).

28 See, for instance, Brown and Stones (1973) and for a more recent account, C. Williams (1994).

29 Davies argues that there is a disjunction between the organisation of nursing work as a series of tasks undertaken by a team of transient workers under the supervision of a skilled nurse, and the professional ideal, that the actual decisions about care are taken by qualified nurses. This leads to feelings of frustration and the fragmentation of patient care (1995: 93–4).

30 Davies argues that nurse managers can do little more than try to make the system work by redeploying staff, finding extra pairs of hands, or exhorting nurses to cope (Davies 1995: 103).

5 THE CONTEMPORARY IMAGINATION

1 The media industries are vertically and horizontally segregated by gender; campaigns for equal opportunities in the workplace were initiated in Britain with the support of the broadcasting unions in the late 1970s, initially achieving some success. For a more detailed account see Baehr and Dyer (1987).

2 White (1985a, 1985b, 1986) provides an account of the post-war period. Rafferty (1992) points to a similar process in the 1930s.

3 For a more detailed account of NHS re-organisation in the 1980s see, for example, Levitt and Wall (1992) and Strong and Robinson (1992).

4 Davies uses the term 'manpower' quite deliberately. Manpower planning was a key element of the strategies put in place by the Committee on Public Accounts

to reduce NHS expenditure, but as Davies points out, the nursing workforce was predominantly female. The assumption, on both the supply and demand sides of manpower planning, is a male career pattern that cannot equally apply to nursing. 'The practices described by manpower planning are the terms in which a discourse of public policy is conducted. It is a discourse which constitutes women's employment as a problem and directs attention away from the devaluing and demeaning dynamics of nursing work' (1995: 88).

5 The UKCC replaced the GNC in 1979 following the Nurses, Midwives and Health Visitors Act, which set up national boards for England, Scotland, Wales and Northern Ireland and the UKCC 'to establish and improve standards of training and professional conduct for nurses, midwives and health visitors' (Nurses, Midwives and Health Visitors Act, S. 2(i), 1979).

6 Davies is a little more circumspect, commenting: 'Six years on, Project 2000 is neither the unqualified success that the optimists would have us believe, nor the "success of the unqualified" that some cynics feared; certainly, however, it falls short of the set of claims that had been initially proposed. Nursing education, by 1990, was on a new footing, but nurse practice remained much as it has always been' (Davies 1995: 126).

7 One of the first strategies used by the professionalisers to detach themselves from other care workers was to establish the right for nurses to define the nature of nursing knowledge. Project 2000 is regarded by its critics as a means of furthering the professional project by re-instituting a hierarchical division of labour between the planners and prescribers of care (who produce care plans and manage their operation) and support workers (who deliver the prescribed care). Critics argue that by adopting the occupational structure of a profession, nurses will become managers and the quality of patient care will decline. The state's apparent support of the new professionalism has to be understood within the context of the decline of the welfare state: see Davies 1995.

8 Buchan and O'May (1998) argue that nursing shortages in the UK are inextricably linked in the minds of the profession and the politicians with pay issues; the unions play the shortage card to argue for pay increases, while the government and the NHS executive play down labour market issues to keep the pressure off the wages bill.

9 The campaign had a specific brief to change the image of nursing: focus group studies amongst fifth and sixth form students revealed that for most young people, nursing meant only general nursing and there was little knowledge or awareness about mental health and mental disability nursing. The profession was still seen as essentially feminine, involving humble jobs and offering no scope for academic satisfaction (Rogers 1984).

10 Trevor Clay points out that the Equal Opportunities Commission had a curious impact on nursing; it focused on making provision for men to train as midwives and ensuring that all recruitment publicity and job advertisements were scrupulously gender-free. Instead of making the NHS a more hospitable working environment for those with family responsibilities, it marginalised what should have been its central concerns (Clay 1987: 118).

11 See, for example, Theodore Dalrymple, 'No wonder her temperature's up', *The Independent*, 20 September 1998.

12 The sample consisted of 410 young people in 21 schools and colleges in urban, suburban and rural catchment areas in the West Midlands and South-East England. See Hemsley-Brown and Foskett 1999.

13 Conversely, ideals of whiteness – blond hair, slim figures and a cult of machismo – encourage young black people to bleach their skin and their hair, and gender

difference is reinforced by the consumption of action series and violent films (Gillespie 1992).

14 Seventy per cent of popular teenage horror aimed at the younger end of the market is produced by Scholastic Productions who additionally produce 'Point Romance', 'Point Detective', 'Point Nurse', 'Sweet Valley High', 'Goose Bumps' and 'Baby-Sitters Club'. The company also publishes educational texts, television programmes, video films, computer software, computer magazines as well as classroom texts and professional magazines (Cooper 1993).

15 Titles include *Katie Goes to College* (1995), *Claire's Conquests* (1995), *Jan's Journey* (1996), *Nikki's New World* (1996), *Nick Finds a Family* (1996), *Barbara's Blues* (1996). All titles published by Scholastic Children's Books, London, a division of Scholastic Ltd, London, New York, Toronto, Sydney, Auckland.

16 Batsford Academic and Educational, 1996.

17 Watts, London, 1996.

18 One of the latest contributions to this growing literature uses content analysis to examine the role of nurses in science fiction. Over 600 books and films are analysed, with results that are very similar to those arrived at through the use of the same methodology to examine images in the past. This creates the impression that there is a timelessness about the ways in which nurses are imagined, that popular fictions reproduce ideologies and values that are unchanging, when, as I argue in this study, the ways in which this repertoire of images are used change historically.

19 A version of this essay appears in Moody and Hallam (1998).

20 Aware of the failures of conventional medical treatment and fed up with the inability of GPs to spend time solving their health problems, many people now turn to alternative therapists and practitioners in an attempt to find someone who will help them manage their illness. A study by the King's Fund shows that, as a nation, we now support more practitioners of complementary and alternative medicine than General Practitioners in a booming industry where female consumers outnumber males by two to one; see the press report by Forma (1997).

21 The creation of Channel 4 in 1982 was a direct response to this remit.

22 For a more detailed discussion, see Hallam and Marshment (1995b).

23 The BBC's charter was reviewed in 1990 with the franchise agreements for independent television and the introduction of new legislation on cable and satellite broadcasting. See Curran and Seaton (1997) for a full account of these changes.

24 For a summary of the controversy see Paul Kerr 1986: 30.

25 In one controversial episode, 'Boiling Point' (27 February 1992), youths set fire to the accident unit. *Casualty* was accused by the veteran clean up TV campaigner Mary Whitehouse of promoting violence; complaints were lodged with the Broadcasting Standards Council, but many viewers wrote in defence of the programme's moral and educative stance. See Hilary Kingsley 1993: 39–42.

26 See, for example, Gerbner, Gross, Morgan and Signorielli (1981).

27 Research consistently shows that British-born women from the Asian diaspora are under-represented amongst nursing students. See Beishon *et al.* (1995) and Iganski *et al.* (1998).

28 In his analysis of nursing discourse, Michael Traynor notes that nursing leaders adapt dominant discourses in their construction of 'professional development', reshaping 'discourse about the profession, the way it is talked about and valued,

in response to changing discourses in society at large ... This can be seen as part of the profession's concern for political and professional power' (1996: 1160).

29 Private nursing homes are employing young women with a minimum of training and support. See S. Thomas, 'Death of innocence', *Guardian Society*, 18 June 1997.

REFERENCES AND
BIBLIOGRAPHY

Abel-Smith, B. (1975) *A History of the Nursing Profession*, London: Heinemann.

Ackroyd, S. (1993) 'Towards an understanding of nurses' attachments to their work: Morale amongst nurses in an acute hospital', *Journal of Advances in Health and Nursing Care* 2, 3: 23–45.

Agbolegbe, G. (1984) 'Fighting the racist disease', *Nursing Times* 80, 6: 18–20.

Alderton, J. (1983) 'The best nurses have the essential qualifications before they go to school. Or do they?', *Nursing Times* 79, 10: 12.

Alexander, S. (1990) 'Working-class terminology and the question of lack', in T. Lovell (ed.) *British Feminist Thought*, Oxford: Blackwell.

Alexander, Z. and Dewjee, A. (eds) (1984) *Wonderful Adventures of Mrs Seacole in Many Lands*, Bristol: Falling Wall Press.

Alley, R.S. (1985) 'Medical melodrama', in B. G. Rose (ed.) *TV Genres: A Handbook and Reference Guide*, Connecticut: Greenwood Press, 73–89.

American Nurse (1982) 'Academy discusses how to improve nursing image', 14,10: 9 and 14.

Anderson, E. (1973) *The Role of the Nurse, Views of the Patient, Nurse and Doctor in some General Hospitals in England*, London: Royal College of Nursing.

Anderson, L. (1980) 'At the threshold of the self: Women and autobiography', in M. Monteith (ed.) *Women's Writing: A Challenge to Theory*, New York: St Martin's Press.

Ansorge, P. (1997) *From Liverpool to Los Angeles: On Writing for Theatre, Film and Television*, London and Boston: Faber and Faber.

Apple, R.D. (1988) 'Image or reality? Photographs in the history of nursing', in A. Hudson Jones (ed.) *Images of Nurses: Perspectives from History, Art and Literature*, Philadelphia: University of Pennsylvania Press.

Ashley, B. (1989) *The Study of Popular Fiction: A Source Book*, London: Pinter Publishers.

Aspinall, S. (1983) 'Women, realism and reality in British films 1943–53', in J. Curran and V. Porter (eds) *British Cinema History*, London: Weidenfeld and Nicolson.

Austin, J.K., Champion, V.L. and Tzeng, O.C.S. (1985) 'Cross-cultural comparison on the nursing image', *International Journal of Nursing Studies* 22, 3: 231–9.

Austin, R. (1976) 'Occupation and Profession in the Organisation of Nursing', unpublished Ph.D. thesis, University College, Cardiff.

—— (1977) 'Sex and gender in the future of nursing', *Nursing Times* Occasional Papers 73, 34: 113–16 and 73, 35: 117–19.

Baehr, H. and Dyer, G. (eds) (1987) *Boxed In: Women in Television*, London: Pandora.

Bailey, P. (1990) 'Parasexuality and glamour: The Victorian barmaid as cultural prototype', *Gender and History* 2, 2: 148–72.

Baker, N. (1989) *Happily Ever After? Women's Fiction in Post-war Britain 1945–60*, London: Macmillan.

Balio, T. (1977) *The American Film Industry*, Madison: University of Wisconsin Press.

Baly, M. (1980) *Nursing and Social Change*, London: Heinemann Medical.

—— (1986) *Florence Nightingale and the Nursing Legacy*, London: Croom Helm.

Banks, J.T. (1988) 'Votaries of life: Patrick White's round-the-clock nurses', in A. Hudson-Jones (ed.) *Images of Nurses*, Philadelphia: University of Pennsylvania Press, 150–71.

Barritt, E.R. (1973) 'Florence Nightingale's values and modern nursing education', *Nursing Forum* 7, 1: 6–47.

Barthes, R. (1973) *Mythologies*, London: Paladin.

Baxter, C. (1988) *The Black Nurse: An Endangered Species. A Case for Equal Opportunities in Nursing*, Cambridge: Training in Health and Race.

Beddoe, D. (1989) *Back to Home and Duty: Women Between the Wars 1918–1939*, London: Pandora.

Beishon, S., Virdee, S. and Hagell, A. (1995) *Nursing in a Multi-Ethnic NHS*, London: Policy Studies Institute.

Bell, C. and Roberts, H. (eds) (1984) *Social Researching: Politics, Problems, Practice*, London: Routledge and Kegan Paul.

Benner, P. (1984) *From Novice to Expert*, California: Addison-Wesley.

Benner, P. and Tanner, C. (1987) 'How expert nurses use intuition', *American Journal of Nursing* 87, 1: 23–31.

Benner, P. and Wrubel, J. (1988) *The Primacy of Caring*, California: Addison-Wesley.

Bennett, T., Martin, C. and Waites, B. (eds) (1982) *Popular Culture: Past and Present*, London: Croom Helm.

Berger, J. (1972) *Ways of Seeing*, Harmondsworth: Penguin.

Bertaux, D. (ed.) (1981) *Biography and Society: The Life History Approach in the Social Sciences*, Newbury Park: Sage Publications.

Betterton, R. (ed.) (1987) *Looking On*, London: Pandora.

Bingham, S. (1980) *Ministering Angels*, London: Van Nos Reinhold.

Birnbaum, D. and Somers, M. (1989) 'The meaning and measurement of occupational image for the nursing role', *Work and Occupations* 16, 2: 200–13.

Bosanquet, N. (ed.) (1979) *Industrial Relations in the NHS: The Search for a System*, London: King Edward's Hospital Fund.

Box, K. and Croft-White, E. (1943) *The Attitudes of Women towards Nursing as a Career*, Central Office of Information, London: HMSO.

Bridges, J.M. (1990) 'Literature review on the images of the nurse and nursing in the media', *Journal of Advanced Nursing* 15: 850–4.

Briggs, A. (1972) *Report of the Briggs Committee on Nursing*, Command 5115, London: HMSO.

Brown, P. and Jordanova, L. (1981) 'Oppressive dichotomies: The nature/culture debate', in E. Whitelegg (ed.) *The Changing Experience of Women*, Milton Keynes: Open University Press.

Brown, R. and Stones, R.W. (1973) *The Male Nurse*, London: Occasional Papers on Social Administration 52, Bell & Sons.

Brownmiller, S. (1986) *Femininity*, London: Paladin/Grafton.

Brunsdon, C. (1991) 'Pedagogies of the feminine: Feminist teaching and women's genres', *Screen* 32, 4: 364–81.

—— (1993) 'Identity in feminist television criticism', *Media, Culture and Society* 15, 2: 309–20.

Bryan, B., Dadzie, S. and Scafe, S. (1985) *The Heart of the Race: Black Women's Lives in Britain*, London: Virago.

Bryman, A. (1992) *Quantity and Quality in Social Research*, London: Routledge.

Buchan, J. and O'May, F. (1998) 'Nursing supply and demand: Reviewing the evidence', *Nursing Times Research* 3, 3: 167–77.

Buchan, J., Waite, R. and Thomas, J. (1989) *Grade Expectations: Clinical Grading and Nurse Mobility*, IMS Report No. 176. Brighton: Institute for Manpower Studies.

Burgess, R.G. (ed.) (1988) *Studies in Qualitative Methodology* Vol. 1, Greenwich, Connecticut: JAI Press Inc.

Butler, J. (1992) 'Contingent foundations: Feminism and the question of "post-modernism"', in J. Butler and J. Scott (eds) *Feminists Theorise the Political*, London: Routledge.

Cadogan, M. and Craig, P. (1976) *You're a Brick, Angela! A New Look at Girls' Fiction from 1839 to 1975*, London: Gollancz.

Cameron, D. (1985) *Feminist Linguistic Theory*, London: Macmillan.

Carpenter, M. (1978) 'Managerialism and the division of labour in nursing', in R. Dingwall and J. Mackintosh (eds) *Readings in the Sociology of Nursing*, Edinburgh: Churchill Livingstone.

—— (1980) 'Asylum nursing before 1914: A chapter in the history of labour', in C. Davies (ed.) *Rewriting Nursing History*, London: Croom Helm.

—— (1990) 'Sex, Class and Race Divisions in Health Care', paper presented at the International Sociological Association Conference 1990.

Carr, H. (1989) *From My Guy to Sci Fi: Genre and Women's Writing in the Postmodern World*, London: Pandora.

Centre for Contemporary Cultural Studies Popular Memory Group (1982) *Making Histories: Studies in History-Writing and Politics*, London: Hutchison.

Chalmers, A.F. (1980) 'Inductivism: Science as knowledge derived from the facts of experience', in A.F. Chalmers, *What Is This Thing Called Science: An Assessment of the Nature and Status of Science and its Methods*, Milton Keynes: Open University Press.

Chanfrault-Duchet, M. (1991) 'Narrative structures, social models, and symbolic representation in the life story', in Sherba B. Gluck and D. Patai (eds) *Women's Words: The Feminist Practice of Oral History*, London: Routledge.

Chapman, C.M. (1977) 'Image of the nurse', *International Nursing Review* 24: 166–70.

Choon, G. and Skevington, S. (1984) 'How do women and men in nursing perceive each other?', in S. Skevington (ed.) *Understanding Nurses*, Chichester: John Wiley and Sons.

Christian-Smith, L.K. (1987) 'Gender, popular culture and curriculum: Adolescent romance novels as gender text', *Curriculum Inquiry* 17, 4: 365–406.

—— (1988) 'Romancing the girl: Adolescent romance novels and the construction of femininity', in L. Roman, L. Christian-Smith and E. Ellsworth (eds) *Becoming Feminine: The Politics of Popular Culture*, London and New York: Falmer Press.

—— (ed.) (1993) *Texts of Desire*, London: Falmer Press.

Chua, Wai Fong and Clegg, S. (1990) 'Professional closure: The case of British nursing', *Theory and Society* 19: 135–72.

Clarke, M. (1976) 'Social Relations Between British and Overseas Student Nurses', unpublished M.Phil. thesis, University of Surrey.

Clay, T. (1987) *Nurses: Power and Politics*, London: Heinemann.

Cleve, L. Van (1988) 'Nursing image as reflected in sex role preferences', *Journal of Nursing Education* 27, 9: 390–3.

Cook, P. (1996) *Fashioning the Nation*, London: British Film Institute.

Cooper, D. (1993) 'Retailing gender: Adolescent book clubs in Australian schools', in L. Christian-Smith (ed.) *Texts of Desire*, London: Falmer Press.

Cope, Z. (1958) *Florence Nightingale and the Doctors*, London: Methuen.

Corradi, C. (1991) 'Text, context and individual meaning: Rethinking life histories in a hermeneutic framework', *Discourse and Society* 2, 1: 105–16.

Cottle, S. (1993) *TV News: Urban Conflict and the Inner City*, Leicester: Leicester University Press.

Couldry, N. (1999) 'Disrupting the media frame at Greenham Common: A new chapter in the history of mediations?', *Media, Culture and Society* 21, 3: 337–58.

Coward, R. (1984) *Female Desire: Women's Sexuality Today*, London: Paladin/Granada.

Cox, M. (1972) 'Problems of overseas nurses training in Britain', *International Nursing Review* 19: 157–68.

Curran, J. and Seaton, J. (1997) *Power Without Responsibility: The Press and Broadcasting in Britain*, London: Routledge.

Dalley, G. (1993) 'The ideological foundations of informal care', in A. Kitson (ed.) *Nursing: Art and Science*, London: Chapman and Hall.

Daniels, T. and Gerson, J. (1989) *The Colour Black: Black Images in British Television*, London: British Film Institute.

Davidoff, L. (1983) 'Class and gender in Victorian England', in J.L. Newton, M.P. Ryan and J.R. Wolkowitz (eds) *Sex and Class in Women's History*, London: Routledge.

Davies, C. (1976) 'Experience of dependency and control in work: The case of nurses', *Journal of Advanced Nursing* 1, 4: 273–82.

—— (1980) *Rewriting Nursing History*, London: Croom Helm.

—— (1988) 'The health visitor as mother's friend: A woman's place in public health 1900–1914', *Social History of Medicine* 1: 39–59.

—— (1995) *Gender and the Professional Predicament in Nursing*, Milton Keynes and Philadelphia: Open University Press.

—— (1996) 'The sociology of professions and the profession of gender', *Sociology* 30, 4: 661–78.

Davies, K., Dickey, J. and Stratford, T. (eds) (1987) *Out of Focus: Writings on Women and the Media*, London: The Women's Press.

Derbyshire, P. (1991) 'Nursing reflections', *Nursing Times* 87, 36: 27–33.

Dickson, N. (1987) 'Best foot forward', *Nursing Times* 83, 1: 39–43.

Dingwall, R. and McIntosh, J. (eds) (1978) *Readings in the Sociology of Nursing*, Edinburgh: Churchill Livingstone.

Dingwall, R., Rafferty, A.M. and Webster, C. (eds) (1988) *An Introduction to the Social History of Nursing*, London: Routledge.

Docherty, D., Morrison, D. and Tracey, M. (1987) *The Last Picture Show? Britain's Changing Film Audiences*, London: British Film Institute.

Douglas, M. (1966) *Purity and Danger: An Analysis of Concepts of Pollution and Taboo*, London: Routledge and Kegan Paul.

Douglas, S. (1995) *Where the Girls Are: Growing up Female with the Mass Media*, London: Penguin.

Doyal, L. (1985) 'Women and the National Health Service: The carers and the careless', in E. Lewin and V. Olesen (eds) *Women Health and Healing: Toward a New Perspective*, London and New York: Tavistock Publications.

Doyal, L., Hunt, G. and Mellor, J. (1981) 'Your life in their hands: Migrant workers in the National Health Service', *Critical Social Policy* 1, 2: 54–71.

Drake, B. (1983) *Women in Trade Unions*, London: Virago.

Drummond, I. and Quinby, L. (1988) *Feminism and Foucault: Reflections on Resistance*, Boston: Northeastern University Press.

Dulewice, S.V. (1970) 'A Study of Nurses' Job Attitudes', unpublished M.Phil. thesis, University of London.

Dunn, A. (1985) *Images of Nursing in the Nursing and Popular Press*, History of Nursing Group, London: Royal College of Nursing.

Dyer, R. (1997) *White*, London: Routledge.

Edwards, R. (1990) 'Connecting method and epistemology: A white woman interviewing black women', *Women's Studies International Forum* 13, 5: 477–90.

Ehrenreich, B. and English, D. (1973) *Witches, Midwives and Nurses: A History of Women Healers*, London: Writers and Readers Publishing Co-operative.

—— (1976) *Complaints and Disorders: The Sexual Politics of Sickness*, London: Writers and Readers Publishing Co-operative.

Ellis, J. (1996) 'The quality film adventure: British cinema critics and the cinema 1942–1948', in A. Higson (ed.) *Dissolving Views: Rethinking British Cinema*, London: Cassell.

Elms, R. and Moorehead, J. (1977) 'Will the "real" nurse please stand up? The stereotype versus reality', *Nursing Forum* 16, 2: 112–27.

Engels, F. (1844/1958) *The Condition of the Working Class in England*, St Albans, Herts: Panther.

Enloe, C. (1983) *Does Khaki Become You? The Militarisation of Women's Lives*, London: Pluto Press.

Evans, M. (1991) *A Good Life: Life at a Girl's Grammar School in the 1950s*, London: Women's Press.

Evers, H. (1981) 'Care or custody? The experiences of women patients in longstay geriatric wards', in B. Hutter and G. Williams (eds) *Controlling Women: The Normal and the Deviant*, London: Croom Helm.

Ewick, P. (1994) 'Integrating feminist epistemologies in undergraduate research methods', *Gender and Society* 8, 1: 92–108.

Fagin, C. and Diers, D. (1983) 'Nursing as metaphor', *New England Journal of Medicine* 309, 2: 116–17.

Farnworth, M. (1958) 'A Study of the Psychological Aspects of the Recruitment of Nurses', unpublished Ph.D. thesis, University of London.

Ferguson, M. (1985) *Forever Feminine: Women's Magazines and the Cult of Femininity*, Hants and Vermont: Gower Publishing.

Fiedler, L.A. (1988) 'Images of the nurse in fiction and popular culture', in A. Hudson Jones (ed.) *Images of Nurses: Perspectives from History, Art and Literature*, Philadelphia: University of Pennsylvania Press.

Finch, J. and Grooves, D. (eds) (1983) *A Labour of Love: Women, Work and Caring*, London: Routledge and Kegan Paul.

Fiske, J. (1987) *Television Culture*, London: Routledge.

Flanagan, M.K. (1982) 'An analysis of nursing as a career choice', in J. Muff (ed.) *Socialisation, Sexism and Stereotyping: Women's Issues in Nursing*, St Louis: C.V. Mosby.

Forma, A. (1997) 'Is therapy making fools of women?', *Independent on Sunday, Real Life*, 2 November: 1–2.

Fowler, B. (1984) 'True to me always: An analysis of women's magazine fiction', in C. Pawling (ed.) *Popular Fiction and Social Change*, London: Macmillan.

—— (1991) *The Alienated Reader: Women and Popular Romantic Literature in the Twentieth Century*, Hemel Hempstead, Herts: Harvester Wheatsheaf.

Francke, L. (1994) *Script Girls*, London: British Film Institute.

Frankenberg, R. (1993) *White Women, Race Matters: The Social Construction of Whiteness*, London: Routledge.

Franklyn, S., Lury, C. and Stacey, J. (1991a) 'Feminism and cultural studies: Pasts, presents and futures', *Media, Culture and Society* 13: 171–92.

—— (eds) (1991b) *Off-Centre: Feminism and Cultural Studies*, London: Harper-Collins.

Freud, S. (1931) 'Female sexuality', in J. Strachey (ed. and trans.) (1953) *Standard Edition of the Complete Psychological Works*, London: Hogarth Press.

Gamarnikow, E. (1978) 'Sexual discrimination of labour: The case of nursing', in A. Kuhn and A. Wolpe (eds) *Feminism and Materialism: Women and Modes of Production*, London: Routledge and Kegan Paul.

—— (1991) 'Nurse or woman: Gender and professionalism in reformed nursing 1860–1923', in P. Holden and J. Littlewood (eds) *Anthropology of Nursing*, London: Routledge.

Gardiner, J.K. (1981) 'On female identity and writing by women', *Critical Inquiry* 8, 2: 347–61.

Gaze, H. (1991) 'Changing images', *Nursing Times* 87, 20: 16–17.

Geiger, S. (1986) 'Women's life histories: Method and content', *Signs* 11, 2: 334–51.

Gerbner, G., Gross, L., Morgan, M. and Signorielli, N. (1981) 'Special report: Health and medicine on television', *The New England Journal of Medicine*, 305.

Giddens, A. (1990) *Modernity and Self-identity: Self and Society in the Late Modern Age*, Cambridge: Polity Press.

Gillespie, M. (1992) *Portrayal of Ethnic Minorities on TV*, London: Research Paper VII, Broadcasting Standards Council Working Paper.

Gilman, S. (1985) *Difference and Pathology: Stereotypes of Sexuality, Race and Madness*, Ithaca: Cornell University Press.

Gilroy, B. (1994) *Black Teacher*, London: Bogle-l'Ouverture Press.

Glazer, N. (1991) '"Between a rock and a hard place": Women's professional organisations in nursing and class, racial and ethnic inequalities', *Gender and Society* 5, 3: 351–72.

Glenn, Evelyn N. (1992) 'From servitude to service work: Historical continuities in the racial division of paid reproductive labour', *Signs* 18, 1: 1–43.

Gluck, Sherna B. and Patai, D. (eds) (1991) *Women's Words: The Feminist Practice of Oral History*, New York and London: Routledge.

Goldsmith, M.L. (1937) *The Woman and the Legend*, London: Hodder and Stoughton.

Graham, H. (1983) 'Caring: A labour of love', in J. Finch and D. Grooves (eds) *A Labour of Love: Women, Work and Caring*, London: Routledge and Kegan Paul.

Griffith, R. (1983) *NHS Management Inquiry*, London: HMSO.

Grosz, E. (1990) 'A note on essentialism and difference', in S. Gunew (ed.) *Feminist Knowledge: Critique and Construct*, London: Routledge.

Gurin, P. and Markus, H. (1989) 'Cognitive consequences of gender identity', in S. Skevington and D. Baker (eds) *The Social Identity of Women*, London/Newbury Park/New Delhi: Sage Publications.

Habenstein, R. and Christ, E. (1955) 'Professionaliser, traditionaliser and utiliser', in G. Mercer (ed.) (1979) *The Employment of Nurses*, London: Croom Helm.

Hall, C. (1979) 'The early formation of Victorian domestic ideology', in S. Burman (ed.) *Fit Work for Women*, London: Croom Helm, 15–33.

Hallam, J. (1996) 'Nursing an image: The *Sue Barton* stories', in S. Sceats and G. Cunningham (eds) *Image and Power: Women in Twentieth Century Fiction*, London: Longmans.

—— (1998) 'Gender and professionalism in TV's medical melodramas', in N. Moody and J. Hallam (eds) *Medical Fictions*, Liverpool: Liverpool John Moores University Press, Association for Research in Popular Fictions.

—— (1999) 'Self image and occupational identity: Barbadian nurses in post-war Britain', in P. Polkey (ed.) *Women's Lives into Print: The Theory, Practice and Writing of Feminist Auto/Biography*, London: Macmillan.

Hallam, J. and Marshall, A. (1993) 'Layers of difference: The significance of a self-reflexive approach for a feminist epistemological project', in M. Kennedy, C. Lubeska and V. Walsh (eds) *Making Connections*, London: Taylor and Francis/Falmer Press.

Hallam, J. and Marshment, M. (1995a) 'Questioning the "ordinary woman": *Oranges are not the Only Fruit*, text and viewer', in B. Skeggs (ed.) *Feminist Cultural Theory: Process and Production*, Manchester: Manchester University Press.

—— (1995b) 'Framing experience: Case studies in reception of *Oranges are not the Only Fruit*', *Screen* 36, 1: 1–15.

Hallam, J. with Marshment, M. (2000) *Realism and Popular Cinema*, Manchester: Manchester University Press.

Halliwell, L. (1989) *Halliwell's Film Guide*, 7th edn, London/New York: Paladin/Grafton.

Hankiss, A. (1981) 'Ontologies of the self: On the mythological rearranging of one's life-history', in D. Bertaux (ed.) *Biography and Society: The Life History Approach in the Social Sciences*, California: Sage Publications.

Hanson, M. and Patchett, T. (1986) 'Nurse recruitment: When the tap runs dry', *Nursing Times* 85, 52: 26–8.

Harding, S. (ed.) (1987) *Feminism and Methodology*, Milton Keynes: Open University Press.

—— (1991) *Whose Science, Whose Knowledge? Thinking from Women's Lives*, Milton Keynes: Open University Press.

Hart, C. (1994) *Behind the Mask: Nurses, Their Unions and Nursing Policy*, London: Balliere Tindall.

Hartsock, N. (1987) 'The feminist standpoint: Developing the ground for a specifically feminist historical materialism', in S. Harding (ed.) *Feminism and Methodology*, Milton Keynes: Open University Press.

Haskell, M. (1974) *From Reverence to Rape: The Treatment of Women in the Movies*, Harmondsworth and Baltimore: Penguin Books Ltd.

Hawkesworth, M.E. (1989) 'Knowers, knowing, known: Feminist theory and claims of truth', *Signs* 14, 3: 533–5.

Hay, G. (1984) 'Recruiting to a price', *Nursing Mirror* 159, 21: 23–6.

Heilbrun, C. (1989) *Writing a Woman's Life*, London: The Women's Press.

Hemsley-Brown, J. and Foskett, N. (1999) 'Career desirability: Young people's perceptions of nursing as a career', *Journal of Advanced Nursing*, 29, 6: 1342–50.

Hermes, J. (1995) *Reading Women's Magazines*, Cambridge: Polity Press.

Heron, L. (ed.) (1985) *Truth, Dare or Promise: Girls Growing Up in the Fifties*, London: Virago.

Hicks, C. (1982) 'Racism in nursing', *Nursing Times* 79: 18–19.

Hill, J. (1985) *Sex, Class and Realism: British Cinema in the 1960s*, London: British Film Institute.

Hockey, L. (1976) *Women in Nursing: A Descriptive Study*, London: Hodder and Stoughton.

Hoëpfl, H. and Hallam, J. (1995) 'The Changing Image of the Nurse: Issues of Identity and Experience', paper presented at IV European Conference on Organisational Psychology and Health Care, Munich.

Holland, K. (1999) 'A journey to becoming: The student nurse in transition', *Journal of Advanced Nursing*, 29, 1: 229–36.

Holloway, J. (1992) 'The media representation of the nurse: The implications for nursing', in K. Soothill, C. Henry and K. Kendrick (eds) *Themes and Perspectives in Nursing*, London: Chapman and Hall.

Holloway, W. (1984) 'Gender difference and the production of subjectivity', in J. Henriques, E. Hollway, C. Urwin, C. Venn and V. Walkerdine (eds) *Changing the Subject: Psychology, Social Regulation and Subjectivity*, London: Methuen.

Hopkins, H. (1963) *The New Look*, London: Secker and Warburg.

Hudson Jones, A. (1988) '*The White Angel* (1936): Hollywood's image of Florence Nightingale', in A. Hudson Jones (ed.) *Images of Nurses: Perspectives from History, Art and Literature*, Philadelphia: University of Pennsylvania Press.

Hughes, L. (1980) 'The public image of the nurse', *Advances in Nursing Science* 2, 3: 55–72.

Hunt, J. (1984) 'Do we deserve our image?', *Nursing Times* 80, 7: 53–5.

Hunter, Kathryn M. (1988) 'Nurses: The satiric image and the translocated ideal', in A. Hudson Jones (ed.) *Images of Nurses: Perspectives from History, Art and Literature*, Philadelphia: University of Pennsylvania Press.

Iganski, P., Mason, D., Humphreys, A. and Watkins, M. (1998) 'The "black" nurse: Ever an endangered species?', *Nursing Times Research* 3, 5: 325–38.

James, W. and Harris, C. (1993) *Inside Babylon: The Caribbean Diaspora in Britain*, London: Verso.

Jarman, F. (1980) 'The Development of Conceptions of Nursing Professionalism among General Hospital Nurses 1860–1895', unpublished Ph.D. thesis, University of Warwick.

Jarrett-Macauley, D. (ed.) (1996) *Reconstructing Womanhood, Reconstructing Feminism: Writings on Black Women*, London: Routledge.

Jeffery, A.J.W. (1950) 'Effects of a Recruitment Film on the Attitudes of School Leavers to Nursing as a Career', unpublished M.Ed. thesis, University of Manchester.

Jelinek, E. (ed.) (1980) *Women's Autobiography: Essays in Criticism*, Bloomington: Indiana University Press.

Jephcott, A.P. (1948) *Rising Twenty*, London: Faber and Faber.

Jones, I.H. (1986) 'Late starters', *Nursing Times* 12, 4: 32–3.

Jones, K. (1967) 'New light on the nursing shortage', *Nursing Times*, 4 August: 1020.

Jordan, M. (1983) '*Carry On*: Follow that stereotype', in J. Curran and V. Porter (eds) *British Cinema History*, London: Weidenfeld and Nicolson.

Jordan, T. (1990) *Growing Up in the Fifties*, London: Macdonald Optima.

Kalisch, B. and Kalisch, P. (1982a) 'Nurses on prime-time television', *American Journal of Nursing* 82, 2: 264–70.

—— (1982b) 'The image of the nurse in motion pictures', *American Journal of Nursing* 82, 4: 605–12.

—— (1982c) 'An analysis of the sources of physician–nurse conflict', in J. Muff (ed.) *Socialisation, Sexism and Stereotyping: Women's Issues in Nursing*, St Louis: C.V. Mosby.

—— (1983) 'Improving the image of nursing', *American Journal of Nursing* 83, 1: 48–55.

—— (1987) *The Changing Image of the Nurse*, California: Addison-Wesley.

Kalisch, B., Kalisch, P. and Scobey, M. (1983) *Images of Nurses on Television*, New York: Springer Publishing Co.

Karpf, A. (1988a) *Doctoring the Media*, London and New York: Routledge.

—— (1988b) 'Broken images', *Nursing Times* 85, 20: 16–17.

Keating, P. (ed.) (1976) *Into Unknown England 1866–1913: Selections from the Social Explorers*, London: Fontana.

Kerr, P. (1986) 'TV and political bias', *The Listener*, 13 November.

Kingsley, H. (1993) *Casualty: The Inside Story*, London: BBC Books.

Kingsley, K. (1988) 'The architecture of nursing', in A. Hudson Jones (ed.) *Images of Nurses: Perspectives from History, Art and Literature*, Philadelphia: University of Pennsylvania Press.

Kreiger, S. (1991) *Social Science and the Self: Personal Essays on an Art Form*, New Jersey: Rutgers University Press.

Kreuger, C. (1978) 'Good girls – bad girls', in R. Dingwall and J. McIntosh (eds) *Readings in the Sociology of Nursing*, Edinburgh: Churchill Livingstone.

Lambeth Council and *The Voice* (1988) *Forty Winters on: Memories of Britain's Postwar Caribbean Immigrants*, London: South London Press.

Lamm, B. (1995) 'Television's forgotten gems: *The Nurses*', *Journal of Popular Film and Television* 23, 2: 72–9.

Lamond, N. (1974) *Becoming a Nurse: The Registered Nurses' View of Student Nurse Education*, London: Royal College of Nursing.

Lancaster, A. (1967) 'A Study of Professional Values and Attitudes among Registered Nurses', unpublished M.Sc. thesis, University of Edinburgh.

Landy, M. (1991) *British Genres: Cinema and Society 1930–1960*, Princeton: Princeton University Press.

de Lauretis, T. (1987) *Technologies of Gender: Essays on Theory, Film and Fiction*, Bloomington: Indiana University Press.

Lawler, J. (1991) *Behind the Screens: Nursing, Somology and the Problem of the Body*, Edinburgh: Churchill Livingstone.

Lawson, M. (1996) 'A clean bill of health', *The Guardian*, 26 June.

Lesbian History Group (eds) (1989) *Not a Passing Phase: Reclaiming Lesbians in History 1840–1985*, London: The Women's Press.

Levitt, R. and Wall, A. (1992) *The Reorganised NHS*, London: Chapman and Hall.

Lewin, E. and Olesen, V. (eds) (1985) *Women Health and Healing: Towards a New Perspective*, London and New York: Tavistock Publications.

Lewis, B.R. (1977a) 'The Marketing of Nursing', unpublished Ph.D. thesis, UMIST, Manchester.

—— (1977b) 'The marketing of nursing as a career', *European Journal of Marketing* 11, 6: 432–44.

Lewis, J. (1992) *Women in Britain since 1945*, Oxford: Blackwell.

Lewis, P. (1978) *The Fifties*, London: Heinemann.

Light, A. (1990) 'Returning to Manderley: Romance fiction, female sexuality and class', in T. Lovell (ed.) *British Feminist Thought*, Oxford: Blackwell.

—— (1991) *Forever England: Femininity, Literature and Conservatism Between the Wars*, London: Routledge.

Littlewood, J. (1991) 'Care and ambiguity: Towards a concept of nursing', in P. Holden and J. Littlewood (eds) *Anthropology of Nursing*, London: Routledge.

Longino, H. (1993) 'Feminist standpoint theory and the problems of knowledge', *Signs* 19, 1: 201–12.

Lovell, M. (1982) 'Daddy's little girl: The lethal effects of paternalism in nursing', in J. Muff (ed.) *Socialisation, Sexism and Stereotyping: Women's Issues in Nursing*, St Louis: C.V. Mosby.

Lury, C. (1991) 'Reading the self: Autobiography, gender and the institution of the literary', in S. Franklin, C. Lury and J. Stacey (eds) *Off-Centre: Feminism and Cultural Studies*, London: HarperCollins.

McClintock, A. (1995) *Imperial Leather: Race, Gender and Sexuality in the Colonial Context*, London: Routledge.

McFarlane, J. (1985) 'Nursing: Images and reality', *Nursing Mirror* 160, 1: 16–18.

MacGuire, J. (1969) *Threshold to Nursing*. Occasional papers on Social Administration 30, London: Bell and Sons Ltd.

Mackay, J. and Thane, P. (1986) 'The Englishwoman', in R. Colls and P. Dodds (eds) *Englishness: Politics and Culture 1880–1920*, London: Croom Helm.

Mackay, L. (1989) *Nursing a Problem*, Milton Keynes: Open University Press.

Maclean, U. (1974) *Nursing in Contemporary Society*, London: Routledge and Kegan Paul.

McMahon, M. (1991) 'Nursing histories: Reviving life in abandoned selves', *Feminist Review* 37: 22–37.

MacNab, G. (1993) *J. Arthur Rank and the British Film Industry*, London and New York: Routledge.

McNay, L. (1992) *Foucault and Feminism*, Cambridge: Polity.

McRobbie, A. (1978) 'Working-class girls and the culture of femininity', in Women's Study Group (eds) *Women Take Issue*, London: Hutchinson.

—— (1982a) 'The politics of feminist research: Between talk, text and action', *Feminist Review* 12: 46–57.

—— (1982b) '*Jackie*: An ideology of adolescent femininity', in T. Bennett, C. Martin and B. Waites (eds) *Popular Culture: Past and Present*, London: Croom Helm.

—— (1991) *Feminism and Youth Culture: From* Jackie *to* Just Seventeen, London: Macmillan.

McRobbie, A. and Nava, M. (1984) *Gender and Generation*, London: Macmillan.

Maggs, C. (1983) *The Origins of General Nursing*, London and Canberra: Croom Helm.

—— (1984) 'Made, not born', *Nursing Times* 80, 38: 31–4.

Mahoney, C. (1997) 'Nice ad. Shame about the reality', *Nursing Times* 93, 6: 12–13.

Maltby, R. (1983) *Harmless Entertainment: Hollywood and the Ideology of Consensus*, Metuchen: Scarecrow Press.

Mama, A. (1995) *Beyond the Masks: Race, Gender and Subjectivity*, London: Routledge.

Mann, P.H. (1974) *A New Survey: The Facts about Romantic Fiction*, London: Mills & Boon.

Marks, S. (1997) 'The legacy of the history of nursing for post-apartheid South Africa', in A.M. Rafferty, J. Robinson and R. Elkan (eds) *Nursing History and the Politics of Welfare*, London: Routledge.

Marshall, H. and Wetherall, M. (1989) 'Talking about career and gender identities: A discourse analysis perspective', in S. Skevington and D. Baker (eds) *The Social Identity of Women*, London/Newbury Park/New Delhi: Sage Publications, 106–29.

Martin, J.L. (1965) 'West Indian pupil nurses and their problems in training', *Nursing Times*, 6 August: 1079–82.

Mascia-Lees, F., Sharpe, P. and Cohen, C.B. (1989) 'The postmodernist turn in anthropology: Cautions from a feminist perspective', *Signs: Journal of Women in Culture and Society* 15, 1: 7–33.

Matz, F. (1969) 'Nurses', in G. Mercer (ed.) (1979) *The Employment of Nurses*, London: Croom Helm.

Melia, K. (1981) 'Student Nurses' Accounts of Their Work and Training: A Qualitative Analysis', unpublished Ph.D. thesis, University of Edinburgh.

—— (1984) 'Student nurses' construction of occupational socialisation', *Sociology of Health and Illness* 6, 2: 132–51.

—— (1987) *Learning and Working: The Occupational Socialisation of Nurses*, London: Tavistock.

Melosh, B. (ed.) (1984) *American Nurses in Fiction*, New York: Garland Press.

—— (1988) '"A special relationship": Nurses and patients in twentieth-century short stories', in A. Hudson Jones (ed.) *Images of Nurses: Perspectives from History, Art and Literature*, Philadelphia: University of Pennsylvania Press.

Mensah, J. (1996) 'Everybody's problem', *Nursing Times* 92, 22: 26–7.

Mercer, G. (ed.) (1979) *The Employment of Nurses: Nursing Labour Turnover in the NHS*, London: Croom Helm.

Milne, P. (1975) 'How six angels were born', *The Listener* 94, 2422: 302–3.

Minghella, E. (1983) 'With angels in mind', *Nursing Times* 79, 34: 45–6.

Modleski, T. (1984) *Loving with a Vengeance: Mass Produced Fantasies for Women*, London and New York: Methuen.

Monteith, M. (ed.) (1986) *Women's Writing: A Challenge to Theory*, New York: St Martin's Press.

Monthly Film Bulletin (1951) 210, 18: 294, 301.

Moody, N. (1998) 'Changing images of medical professionalism in the *Star Trek* universe', in N. Moody and J. Hallam (eds) *Medical Fictions*, Liverpool: Liverpool John Moores University and the Association for Research in Popular Fictions.

Moody, N. and Hallam, J. (eds) (1998) *Medical Fictions*, Liverpool: Liverpool John Moores University and the Association for Research in Popular Fictions.

Morley, D. (1986) *Family Television*, London: Comedia.

—— (1992) *Television, Audiences and Cultural Studies*, London: Routledge.

Morton-Williams, J. and Berthoud, R. (1971) *Nurses Attitude Study: Report on Postal Survey*, London: Social Community Planning and Research.

Muff, J. (1982a) 'Altruism, socialism, and nightingalism: The compassion traps', in J. Muff (ed.) *Socialisation, Sexism and Stereotyping: Women's Issues in Nursing*, St Louis: C.V. Mosby.

—— (1982b) 'Handmaiden, battleaxe, whore: An exploration into the fantasies, myths and stereotypes about nurses', in J. Muff (ed.) *Socialisation, Sexism and Stereotyping: Women's Issues in Nursing*, St Louis: C.V. Mosby.

—— (1988) 'Of images and ideals: A look at socialisation and sexism in nursing', in A. Hudson Jones (ed.) *Images of Nurses: Perspectives from History, Art and Literature*, Philadelphia: University of Pennsylvania Press.

Mulvey, L. (1975) 'Visual pleasure and narrative cinema', *Screen* 16, 3: 6–18.

Murphy, R. (1983) 'Rank's attempt on the American market 1944–49', in J. Curran and V. Porter (eds) *British Cinema History*, London: Weidenfeld and Nicolson.

—— (1989) *Realism and Tinsel: Cinema and Society in Britain 1939–49*, London and New York: Routledge.

Myrdal, A. and Klein, V. (1956) *Women's Two Roles*, London: Routledge and Kegan Paul.

Nead, L. (1988) *Myths of Sexuality: Representations of Women in Victorian Britain*, Oxford: Blackwell.

Neagle, A. (1958) 'Portraying Edith Cavell and other nurses', *Nursing Mirror* 10: 1–11.

Nuffield Provincial Hospitals Trust (1953) *The Work of Nurses in Hospital Wards*, Nuffield Provincial Hospitals Trust, London.

Oakley, A. (1980) 'Interviewing women: A contradiction in terms', in H. Roberts (ed.) *Doing Feminist Research*, London: Routledge and Kegan Paul.

—— (1984) 'The importance of being a nurse', *Nursing Times* 80, 50: 26.

Ogier, Margaret E. (1982) *An Ideal Sister? A Study of the Leadership Style and Verbal Interactions of Ward Sisters with Nurse Learners in General Hospitals*, London: Royal College of Nursing.

Owens, P. and Glennerster, H. (1990) *Nursing in Conflict*, London: Macmillan.

Paizis, G. (1998) *Love and the Novel: The Poetics and Politics of Romantic Fiction*, London: Macmillan.

Palfrey, C. (1989) 'Public perceptions of nursing', *Nursing Times* 85, 36: 54.

Patterson, S. (1963) *Dark Strangers: A Sociological Study of the Absorption of a Recent West Indian Migrant Group in Brixton, South London*, London: Tavistock.

Patton, M. (1987) *How to Use Qualitative Methods in Evaluation*, Newbury Park: Sage.

Pavey, A. (1938) *The Story of the Growth of Nursing*, London: Faber.

Pawling, C. (1984) *Popular Fiction and Social Change*, London: Macmillan.

Pearce, L. and Stacey, J. (eds) (1995) *Romance Revisited*, New York: New York University Press.

Pearson, A. (1983) 'What the public thinks', *Nursing Times* 79, 8: 18–19.

Personal Narratives Group (eds) (1989) *Interpreting Women's Lives, Feminist Theory and Personal Narratives*, Bloomington and Indianapolis: Indiana University Press.

Pfau, M., Mullen, L.J. and Garrow, K. (1995) 'The influence of television viewing on public perceptions of physicians', *Journal of Broadcasting and Electronic Media*, 39: 441–58.

Philips, D. (1998) 'Healthy heroines: Sue Barton, Lillian Wald, Lavinia Lloyd Dock and the Henry Street Settlement', *Journal of American Studies* 33, 1: 65–82.

Platt, J. (1988) 'What can case studies do?' in R.G. Burgess (ed.) *Studies in Qualitative Methodology* Vol. 1, Greenwich, Connecticut: JAI Press, 1–23.

Plummer, K. (1983) *Documents of Life: An Introduction to the Problems and Literature of Humanistic Method*, London: Allen and Unwin.

Pomeranz, R. (1973) *The Lady Apprentices: A Study of Transition in Nurse Training*, Occasional Papers on Social Administration 51, London: Bell and Sons Ltd.

Poovey, M. (1984) *The Proper Lady and the Woman Writer: Ideology as Style in the Works of Mary Wollstonecraft, Mary Shelley and Jane Austen*, Chicago: University of Chicago Press.

—— (1989) *Uneven Developments: The Ideological Work of Gender in Mid-Victorian England*, London: Virago.

Porter, S. (1992) 'The poverty of professionalisation: A critical analysis of strategies for the occupational advancement of nursing', *Journal of Advanced Nursing* 17: 720–6.

Press, A. (1991) *Women Watching Television: Gender, Class and Generation in the American Television Experience*, Philadelphia: University of Pennsylvania Press.

Preston, A. (1990) 'The invisible woman: Two decades of magazine images of nurses', *Journal of Communications*, Winter: 48–60.

Probyn, E. (1993) *Sexing the Self: Gendered Positions in Cultural Studies*, London and New York: Routledge.

Radstone, S. (ed.) (1988) *Sweet Dreams: Sexuality, Gender and Popular Fiction*, London: Lawrence and Wishart.

Radway, J. (1984) *Reading the Romance: Women, Patriarchy and Popular Literature*, Chapel Hill and London: University of North Carolina Press.

Rafferty, A.M. (1992) 'Nursing policy and the nationalisation of nursing: The representation of "crisis" and the "crisis" of representation', in J. Robinson, A. Gray and R. Elkan (eds) *Policy Issues in Nursing*, Milton Keynes: Open University Press.

Randall, R.S. (1977) 'Censorship: From *The Miracle* to *Deep Throat*', in T. Balio (ed.) *The American Film Industry*, Madison: University of Wisconsin Press.

Ray, S. (1974) *Children's Fiction: A Handbook for Librarians*, Leicester: Brockhampton Press.

Reynolds, K. (1996) *Young People's Reading at the End of the Century*, London: Book Trust.

Richardson, H. (1988) 'Uniform appeal', *Nursing Times* 84, 24: 46–7.

Roberts, E. (1986) *A Woman's Place*, Oxford: Blackwell.

—— (1995) *Women and Families: An Oral History 1940–1970*, Oxford: Blackwell.

Robinson, J., Gray, A. and Elkan, R. (eds) (1992) *Policy Issues in Nursing*, Milton Keynes: Open University Press.

Rogers, R. (1984) 'The image makers', *Senior Nurse* 1, 6: 10–11.

Roman, L.G., Christian-Smith, L.K. and Ellsworth, E. (eds) (1988) *Becoming Feminine: The Politics of Popular Culture*, London: Falmer Press.

Roots Oral History (1992) *Rude Awakening: African/Caribbean Settlers in Manchester*, Manchester: Roots Oral History Project.

Roper, N. (1976) 'An image of nursing for the 1970s', *Nursing Times* 72, 17: 61–4.

Ross, K. (1996) *Black and White Media: Black Images in Popular Film and Television*, Cambridge: Polity.

Rowbotham, J. (1989) *Good Girls Make Good Wives: Guidance for Girls in Victorian Fiction*, Oxford: Basil Blackwell.

Royal College of Nursing (1992) *The Value of Nursing*, London: Royal College of Nursing.

Rushcliffe, H.B.B. (1945) Report of the Committee on the Training of Nurses for the Colonies, London: HMSO.

Salvage, J. (1982) 'Angles, not angels', *Health Services Journal* 3, 9: 12–13.

—— (1983a) 'Distorted images', *Nursing Times* 79, 1: 13–15.

—— (1983b) 'Changing the image', *International Nursing Review* 30, 6.

—— (1985) *The Politics of Nursing*, London: Heinemann.

—— (1987a) *Nurses, Gender and Sexuality*, London: Heinemann.

—— (1987b) 'We're no angels – images of nurses', in K. Davies, J. Dickey and T. Stratford (eds), *Out of Focus: Writings on Women in the Media*, London: The Women's Press.

—— (1992) 'The new nursing', in J. Robinson, A. Gray and R. Elkan (eds) *Policy Issues in Nursing*, Milton Keynes: Open University Press.

Sceats, S. and Cunningham, G. (eds) (1996) *Image and Power: Women in Twentieth Century Fiction*, London: Longmans.

Scott, H. (1997) 'New nursing stereotype depicts nurses as thick', *British Journal of Nursing* 6, 8.

Seccombe, I., Jackson, C. and Patch, A. (1995) *Nursing: The Next Generation*, Sussex: IES Report 274.

Sheridan, D. (1990) 'Ambivalent memories: Women and the 1939–45 war in Britain', *Oral History*, Spring: 32–9.

Shields, Vickie R. and Dervin, B. (1993) 'Sense-making in feminist social science research: A call to enlarge the methodological options of feminist studies', *Women's Studies International Forum* 16, 1: 65–81.

Silverstone, R. (1994) *Television and Everyday Life*, London: Routledge.

Simnett, A. (1986) 'The pursuit of respectability: Women and the nursing profession 1860–1900', in R. White (ed.) *Political Issues in Nursing: Past, Present and Future*, Vol. 2, Chichester: John Wiley and Sons Ltd.

Simpson, H.M. (1977) 'The Royal College of Nursing of the United Kingdom 1916–1976: Role and action in a changing health service', *Journal of Advanced Nursing* 2: 281–98.

Singh, A. (1970) 'The student nurse on experimental courses – attitudes towards nursing as a career', *International Journal of Nursing Studies*, 7: 201–24.

Skeggs, B. (ed.) (1995) *Feminist Cultural Theory: Process and Production*, Manchester: Manchester University Press.

—— (1997) *Formations of Class and Gender: Becoming Respectable*, London/Newbury Park/New Delhi: Sage.

Skevington, S. (ed.) (1984) *Understanding Nurses: The Social Psychology of Nursing*, Chichester: John Wiley and Sons.

Skevington, S. and Baker, D. (eds) (1989) *The Social Identity of Women*, London/Newbury Park/New Delhi: Sage Publications.

Smith, D. (1988a) *The Everyday World as Problematic: A Feminist Sociology*, Milton Keynes: Open University Press.

—— (1988b) 'Femininity as discourse', in L. Roman, L. Christian-Smith and E. Ellsworth (eds) *Becoming Feminine: The Politics of Popular Culture*, London: Falmer Press.

Smith, F.B. (1982) *Florence Nightingale: Reputation and Power*, London: Croom Helm.

Smith, P. (1992) *The Emotional Labour of Nursing: How Nurses Care*, Basingstoke: Macmillan.

Snape, D., Thompson, K. and Chetwynd, M. (1995) *Discrimination Against Gay Men and Lesbians: A Study of the Nature and Extent of Discriminations Against Homosexual Men and Women in Britain Today*, London: Social and Community Planning Research.

Snitow, A. (1984) 'Mass market romance: Pornography for women is different', in A. Snitow, C. Stansell and S. Thomson (eds) *Desire: The Politics of Sexuality*, London: Virago.

Spence, J. (1986) *Putting Myself in the Picture: A Political, Personal and Photographic Autobiography*, London: Camden Press.

Stacey, J. (1994) *Star Gazing: Hollywood Cinema and Female Spectatorship*, London: Routledge.

Stacey, M. (1988) *The Sociology of Health and Healing*, London/Boston: Unwin Hyman.

Stanley, L. (ed.) (1984) *The Diaries of Hannah Cullwick*, London: Virago.

—— (ed.) (1990a) *Feminist Praxis: Research, Theory and Epistemology in Feminist Sociology*, London: Routledge

—— (1990b) 'Moments of writing: Is there a feminist auto/biography?' *Gender and History* 2, 1: 58–67.

Starkey, P. (ed.) (1994) *Nursing Memories from Probationers to Professors*, Liverpool: National Museums and Galleries on Merseyside.

Steedman, C. (1986) *Landscape for a Good Woman: A Story of Two Lives*, London: Virago.

—— (1989) 'Women's biography and autobiography: Forms of history, histories of form', in H. Carr (ed.) *From My Guy to Sci Fi: Genre and Women's Writing in the Postmodern World*, London: Pandora.

—— (1992) *Past Tenses: Essays on Writing, Autobiography and History*, London: Rivers Oram Press.

Stein, L. (1967) 'The doctor–nurse game', *Archives of General Psychology* 16: 699–703.

Stein, L., Watts, D. and Howell, T. (1990) 'The doctor–nurse game revisited', *New England Journal of Medicine*, 322, 8: 546–9.

Stones, R.W.H. (1972) 'Overseas nurses in Britain: A study of male recruits', *Nursing Times* 9, 7: 141–4.

Strauss, A. and Corbin, J. (1990) *Basics of Qualitative Research: Grounded Theory Procedures and Techniques*, London: Sage.

Strong, P. and Robinson, J. (1992) *The NHS – Under New Management*, Milton Keynes and Philadelphia: Open University Press.

Summers, A. (1983) 'Pride and prejudice: Ladies and nurses in the Crimean War', *History Workshop* 16: 33–56.

—— (1988) *Angels and Citizens: British Women as Military Nurses 1854–1914*, London: Routledge and Kegan Paul.

Tattam, A. (1989) 'Misleading image?' *Nursing Times* 85, 10: 22.

Taylor, H. (1989) 'Romantic readers', in H. Carr (ed.) *From My Guy to Sci Fi: Genre and Women's Writing in the Postmodern World*, London: Pandora.

Taylor, J. (1982) 'Picturing the past: Documentary realism in the 1930s', *Ten 8*, 11.

Thackery, R. (1999) 'Fast track: Carry on nursing, please: We need nurses but it seems nobody wants to be one. Except a new breed of highly articulate graduates', *The Independent*, 28 January.

Thomas, M. and Morton-Williams, J. (1972) *Overseas Nurses in Britain. Evidence to the Briggs Committee on Nursing*, London: P.E.P. Broadsheet 539.

Thompson, P. (1981) 'Life histories and the analysis of social change', in D. Bertaux (ed.) *Biography and Society*, Newbury Park: Sage Publications.

Thompson, S. (1974) 'Overseas nurses deserve better protection', *New Psychiatry* 9, 3: 22–3.

Thumim, J. (1992) *Celluloid Sisters: Women and Popular Cinema*, London: Macmillan.

Tinkler, P. (1995) *Constructing Girlhood: Popular Magazines for Girls Growing Up in England 1920–1950*, London: Taylor and Francis.

Torkington, P. (1985) 'Racism in the National Health Service: A Liverpool Profile', unpublished Ph.D. thesis, University of Liverpool.

Toynbee, P. (1983) 'The ladies no longer have lamps', *World Medicine*, 18, 11: 32.

Traynor, M. (1996) 'Looking at discourse in a literature review of nursing texts', *Journal of Advanced Nursing* 23: 1155–61.

Treacher, A. (1988) 'What is life without my love? Desire and romantic fiction', in S. Radstone (ed.) *Sweet Dreams: Sexuality, Gender and Popular Fiction*, London: Lawrence and Wishart.

Truman, C. (1987) 'Managing the career-break', *Nursing Times* 83, 3: 44–5.

Turow, J. (1989) *Playing Doctor: Television, Storytelling and Medical Power*, Milton Keynes: Open University Press.

UK Council for Overseas Student Affairs (1971) *Overseas Nurses in Britain. Evidence to the Briggs Committee on Nursing 1972*, London: UKCOSA.

Vicinus, M. (1977) *Suffer and Be Still: Women in the Victorian Age*, Bloomington and London: Indiana University Press.

—— (1985) *Independent Women: Work and Community for Single Women 1850–1920*, London: Virago.

Vicinus, M. and Nergaard, B. (eds) (1989) *Ever Yours, Florence Nightingale. Selected Letters*, London: Virago.

Vousden, M. (1988) 'Please put your son in the ward, Mrs Worthington', *Nursing Times* 84, 15: 35–6.

—— (1989a) 'Selling nursing – value for money?', *Nursing Times* 85, 34: 25–9.

—— (1989b) 'Selling nursing – analysing the response', *Nursing Times* 85, 35: 47–8.

Walby, S. and Greenwell, J. with Mackay, L. and Soothill, K. (1994) *Medicine and Nursing: Professions in a Changing Health Service*, London/Newbury Park/New Delhi: Sage.

Walkerdine, V. (1990) *Schoolgirl Fictions*, London: Verso.

Ware, V. (1992) *Beyond the Pale: White Women, Racism and History*, London: Verso.

Warr, J. (1996) 'Vocationalism: A mirror on the profession', *Nurse Education Today* 16: 267–9.

—— (1998) 'An evaluative study into the effectiveness of level 3 NVQ support staff to nurses', *Nurse Education Today*, 18: 505–16.

Webster, W. (1998) *Imagining Home: Gender, Race and National Identity, 1945–64*, London: UCL Press.

West, M. and Rushton, R. (1986) 'The drop-out factor', *Nursing Times* 82, 52: 29–31.

White, R. (1985a) *The Effects of the NHS on the Nursing Profession 1948–61*, London: King's Fund.

—— (1985b) 'Political regulators in British nursing', in R. White (ed.) *Political Issues in Nursing: Past, Present and Future*, Vol. 1, Chichester: John Wiley and Sons.

—— (1986) 'From matron to manager: The political construction of reality', in R. White (ed.) *Political Issues in Nursing: Past, Present and Future*, Vol. 2, Chichester: John Wiley and Sons.

Whittaker, E. and Olesen, V. (1984) 'The faces of Florence Nightingale: Functions of the heroine legend in an occupational sub-culture', *Human Organisation* 23, 1: 123–30.

Williams, A. (1990) 'Reflections on the making of an ethnographic text', *Studies in Sexual Politics* 29: 1–63.

Williams, C. (1994) 'Men in Nursing: On the Glass Elevator, Lazy or Gay?', paper presented at the British Sociological Association Conference, Preston.

Williams, (Ysgafell) J. (1987) *An Autobiography of Elizabeth Davis. Betsy Cadwaladyr: A Balaclava Nurse*, Cardiff: Honno.

Williams, K. (1978) 'Ideologies of nursing: Their meanings and implications', in R. Dingwall and J. McIntosh (eds) *Readings in the Sociology of Nursing*, Edinburgh: Churchill Livingstone.

Williams, R. (1963) *Culture and Society, 1780–1950*, Harmondsworth: Penguin.

—— (1977) *Marxism and Literature*, Oxford: Oxford University Press.

Williamson, V. (1998) 'Labour of love: Gender and the delivery of the nineties Mills & Boon medical', in N. Moody and J. Hallam (eds) *Medical Fictions*, Liverpool: Liverpool John Moores University and the Association for Research in Popular Fictions.

Wilson, E. (1980) *Only Halfway to Paradise: Women in Postwar Britain 1945–68*, London and New York: Tavistock.

—— (1988) 'Tell it like it is: Women and confessional writing', in S. Radstone (ed.) *Sweet Dreams: Sexuality, Gender and Popular Fiction*, London: Lawrence and Wishart.

Witz, A. (1992) *Professions and Patriarchy*, London: Routledge.

Young, A. (1990) *Femininity in Dissent*, London: Routledge.

Young, L. (1996) *Fear of the Dark: 'Race', Gender and Sexuality in the Cinema*, London: Routledge.

INDEX

CPSIA information can be obtained at www.ICGtesting.com
Printed in the USA
LVOW10s2352210214

374565LV00002B/16/P